Lecture Notes in Computer Science   8678

Commenced Publication in 1973
Founding and Former Series Editors:
Gerhard Goos, Juris Hartmanis, and Jan van Leeuwen

T0219714

Cristian A. Linte   Ziv Yaniv
Pascal Fallavollita   Purang Abolmaesumi
David R. Holmes III (Eds.)

Augmented Environments for Computer-Assisted Interventions

9th International Workshop, AE-CAI 2014
Held in Conjunction with MICCAI 2014
Boston, MA, USA, September 14, 2014
Proceedings

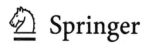 Springer

Volume Editors

Cristian A. Linte
Rochester Institute of Technology
Rochester, NY, USA
E-mail: clinte@mail.rit.edu

Ziv Yaniv
Children's National Health System
Washington, DC, USA
E-mail: zyaniv@childrensnational.org

Pascal Fallavollita
Technical University of Munich, Germany
E-mail: fallavol@in.tum.de

Purang Abolmaesumi
University of British Columbia
Vancouver, BC, Canada
E-mail: purang@ece.ubc.ca

David R. Holmes III
Mayo Clinic, Rochester, MN, USA
E-mail: holmes.david3@mayo.edu

ISSN 0302-9743   e-ISSN 1611-3349
ISBN 978-3-319-10436-2   e-ISBN 978-3-319-10437-9
DOI 10.1007/978-3-319-10437-9
Springer Cham Heidelberg New York Dordrecht London

Library of Congress Control Number: 2014946280

LNCS Sublibrary: SL 6 – Image Processing, Computer Vision, Pattern Recognition, and Graphics

Typesetting: Camera-ready by author, data conversion by Scientific Publishing Services, Chennai, India

Printed on acid-free paper

Springer is part of Springer Science+Business Media (www.springer.com)

Preface

Welcome to the 9th edition of the Augmented Reality for Computer-Assisted Interventions (AE-CAI) workshop. We are pleased to present the proceedings of this exciting workshop held in conjunction with MICCAI 2014 on September 14, 2014 in Boston, Massachusetts, USA.

The event was jointly organized by scientists from Rochester Institute of Technology (Rochester, NY, USA), Children's National Health System (Washington, DC, USA), Technical University of Munich (Munich, Germany), University of British Columbia (Vancouver, BC, Canada), and Mayo Clinic (Rochester, MN, USA), who have had a long-standing tradition in the development and application of augmented and virtual environments for medical imaging and image-guided interventions. In addition, a Program Committee consisting of more than 70 international experts served as reviewers for the submitted papers.

Rapid technical advances in medical imaging, including its growing applications to drug delivery and minimally invasive/interventional procedures, as well as a symbiotic development of imaging modalities, and nano-technological devices, have attracted significant interest in recent years. This has been fueled by the clinical and basic science research endeavors to obtain more detailed physiological and pathological information about the human body, to facilitate the study of localized genesis and progression of diseases. Current research has also been motivated by the development of medical imaging from being a primarily diagnostic modality toward its role as a therapeutic and interventional aid, driven by the need to streamline the diagnostic and therapeutic processes via minimally invasive visualization and therapy.

The objective of the AE-CAI workshop was to attract scientific contributions that offer solutions to the technical problems in the area of augmented and virtual environments for computer-assisted interventions, and to provide a venue for dissemination of papers describing both complete systems and clinical applications. The community also encourages a broad interpretation of the field - from macroscopic to molecular imaging, passing the information on to scientists and engineers for the development of breakthrough therapeutics, diagnostics, and medical devices, which can then be seamlessly delivered back to patients. The workshop attracted researchers in computer science, biomedical engineering, computer vision, robotics, and medical imaging. This meeting featured a single track of oral and poster presentations showcasing original research engaged in the development of virtual and augmented environments for medical image visualization and image-guided interventions.

In addition to the proffered papers and posters, we were pleased to welcome as keynote speakers Dr. Guang-Zhong Yang (Imperial College London, London, UK), speaking on the integration of medical robotics and computer vision for computer-assisted interventions, and Dr. Craig Peters (Children's National

Health System, Washington, DC, USA), describing state-of-the-art developments in patient-based augmented environments for pediatric minimally invasive interventions and robotic surgery.

AE-CAI 2014 attracted 23 paper submissions from eight countries. The submissions were distributed for review to the Program Committee and each paper was evaluated, in a double-blind manner, by at least three experts, who provided detailed critiques and constructive comments to the authors and workshop editorial board. Based on the reviews, 15 papers were selected for oral and poster presentation and publication in these proceedings. The authors revised their submissions according to the reviewers' suggestions, and resubmitted their manuscripts, along with their response to reviewers, for a final review by the volume editors (to ensure that all reviewers' comments were properly addressed) prior to publication in this collection.

On behalf of the AE-CAI 2014 Organizing Committee, we would like to extend our sincere thanks to all Program Committee members for providing detailed and timely reviews of the submitted manuscripts. We also thank all authors, presenters, and attendees at AE-CAI 2014 for their scientific contribution, enthusiasm, and support. We hope that you all will enjoy reading this volume and we look forward to your continuing support and participation in our next AE-CAI event to be hosted at MICCAI 2015 in Munich, Germany.

July 2014

Cristian A. Linte
Ziv Yaniv
Pascal Fallavollita
Purang Abolmaesumi
David R. Holmes III

AE-CAI 2014 Workshop Committees

Organizing Committee

Cristian A. Linte	Rochester Institute of Technology, USA
Ziv Yaniv	Children's National Health System, USA
Pascal Fallavollita	Technical University of Munich, Germany
Purang Abolmaesumi	University of British Columbia, Canada
David R. Holmes III	Mayo Clinic, Rochester, USA

Program Committee

Takehiro Ando	The University of Tokyo, Japan
Leon Axel	NYUMC, USA
Adrien Bartoli	ISIT, UK
John Baxter	Robarts Research Institute, Canada
Marie-Odile Berger	Inria, France
Wolfgang Birkfellner	MU Vienna, Austria
Tobias Blum	Technische Universität München, Germany
Yiyu Cai	Nanyang Technological University, Singapore
Cheng Chen	University of Bern, Switzerland
Chung-Ming Chen	National Taiwan University, Taiwan
Elvis Chen	Robarts Research Institute, Canada
Xinjian Chen	Soochow University, Taiwan
Kevin Cleary	Children's National Medical Center, USA
Louis Collins	McGill University, Canada
Simon Drouin	McGill University, Canada
Eddie Edwards	Imperial College, UK
Gary Egan	University of Melbourne, Australia
Yong Fan	Institute of Automation, Chinese Academy of Sciences, China
Gabor Fichtinger	Queen's University, Canada
Michael Figl	Medical University of Vienna, Austria
Kenko Fujii	Imperial College, UK
John Galeotti	Carnegie Mellon University, USA
James Gee	University of Pennsylvania, USA
Stamatia Giannarou	Imperial College London, UK
Ali Gooya	University of Pennsylvania, USA
Lixu Gu	Shanghai Jiaotong University, China
Makoto Hashizume	Kyushu University, Japan
David Hawkes	University College London, UK

Jaesung Hong	Daegu Gyeongbuk Institute of Science and Technology, South Korea
Robert D. Howe	Harvard University, USA
Pierre Jannin	Université de Rennes I, France
Bernhard Kainz	Imperial College London, UK
Ali Kamen	Siemens Corporate Research, USA
Ron Kikinis	Harvard and SPL, USA
Jan Klein	Fraunhofer MEVIS, Germany
David Kwartowitz	Clemson University, USA
Rudy Lapeer	University of East Anglia, UK
Su-Lin Lee	Imperial College, UK
Ming Li	National Institutes of Health, USA
Jimmy Liu	Agency for Science, Technology and Research, Singapore
Tianming Liu	UGA, USA
Gian-Luca Mariottini	University Texas at Arlington, USA
John Moore	Robarts Research Institute, Canada
Kensaku Mori	Nagoya University, Japan
Ryoichi Nakamura	Chiba University, Japan
Nassir Navab	Technische Universität München, Germany
Philip Pratt	Imperial College London, UK
Maryam Rettmann	Mayo Clinic, USA
Jannick Rolland	University of Rochester, USA
Ichiro Sakuma	The University of Tokyo, Japan
Yoshinobu Sato	Nara Institute of Science and Technology, Japan
Julia Schnabel	University of Oxford, UK
Dinggang Shen	UNC, USA
Pengcheng Shi	Rochester Institute of Technology, USA
Amber Simpson	Vanderbilt University, USA
George Stetten	University of Pittsburgh/CMU, USA
Danail Stoyanov	University College London, UK
Russell H. Taylor	Johns Hopkins University, USA
Tamas Ungi	Queen's University, Canada
Theo Van Walsum	Erasmus MC, The Netherlands
Kirby Vosburgh	BWH/Harvard, USA
Guangzhi Wang	Tsinghua University, China
Jaw-Lin Wang	National Taiwan University, Taiwan
Junchen Wang	The University of Tokyo, Japan
Stefan Wesarg	Fraunhofer IGD, Germany
Kelvin K. Wong	Methodist Hospital - Weill Cornell Medical College, USA

Table of Contents

Graphics Processor Unit (GPU) Accelerated Shallow Transparent Layer Detection in Optical Coherence Tomographic (OCT) Images for Real-Time Corneal Surgical Guidance

Tejas Sudharshan Mathai[1,2], John Galeotti[1,2],
Samantha Horvath[2], and George Stetten[1,2]

[1] Department of Biomedical Engineering, Carnegie Mellon University, Pittsburgh, USA
[2] Robotics Institute, Carnegie Mellon University, Pittsburgh, USA
tmathai@andrew.cmu.edu

Abstract. An image analysis algorithm is described that utilizes a Graphics Processor Unit (GPU) to detect in real-time the most shallow subsurface tissue layer present in an OCT image obtained by a prototype SDOCT corneal imaging system. The system has a scanning depth range of 6mm and can acquire 15 volumes per second at the cost of lower resolution and signal-to-noise ratio (SNR) than diagnostic OCT scanners. To the best of our knowledge, we are the first to experiment with non-median percentile filtering for simultaneous noise reduction and feature enhancement in OCT images, and we believe we are the first to implement any form of non-median percentile filtering on a GPU. The algorithm was applied to five different test images. On an average, it took ~0.5 milliseconds to preprocess an image with a 20th-percentile filter, and ~1.7 milliseconds for our second-stage algorithm to detect the faintly imaged transparent surface.

Keywords: OCT, image-guidance, real-time, GPU, percentile filter, surface detection.

1 Introduction

Spectral Domain Optical Coherence Tomography (SDOCT) is a non-invasive, non-contact imaging modality that has found great use in ophthalmology for corneal and retinal disease diagnosis. SDOCT uses near-infrared wavelengths, typically in the 800nm-1600nm range, to image sub-surface structures - including transparent surfaces - in soft tissue, such as those in the anterior segment of the eye and the retina. These light waves penetrate not only the clear cornea and lens, but also the opaque limbus, where important physiological processes take place at the intersection of the cornea, iris, and sclera. The basic acquisition unit of a SDOCT scanner is a one-dimensional axial scan (*A-scan*) along the beam path, but by rapidly steering the OCT beam, multiple A-scans can be combined to produce 2-D and 3-D high resolution cross-sectional images of the tissue. [1, 2] Over the past few years, there has been

C.A. Linte et al. (Eds.): AE-CAI 2014, LNCS 8678, pp. 1–13, 2014.

significant progress towards the creation of SDOCT systems that provide higher image acquisition speeds. Since OCT was first demonstrated in 1991, the A-scan rates have gone up from 400 Hz to 20 MHz in experimental systems. [3] Most of the commercially available SDOCT systems operate using line scan rates within 30 – 85 KHz to produce high quality 2D *B-scan* images. The fastest spectrometer-based SDOCT systems that have been developed operate with a dual camera configuration and a 500 KHz A-scan rate. [4] These SDOCT setups have been used to obtain 2D images and 3D volumes; for high resolution 3D volumetric scans, the acquisition time is still on the order of seconds. [5, 6, 7] However, most of the SDOCT systems today were developed for diagnosis rather than clinical surgery, and only a few attempts have been made to integrate real-time OCT into eye surgery. OCT systems have been previously combined with surgical microscopes in order to obtain cross-sections of the sclera and cornea, but these systems were used in a "stop and check" scenario rather than for real-time guidance. [8, 9] It is a challenge to integrate a SDOCT system into interactive eye surgery while satisfying clinicians' needs and preferences for high resolution, high signal-to-noise ratio (SNR), and real-time frame rates. In order to produce higher resolution images, more samples of the target need to be acquired, and higher contrast images with better SNR require a longer exposure for each individual A-scan (longer dwell time at each spot on the target). [2] SDOCT images are inevitably affected by noise. [11-14] A tradeoff always exists between fast image acquisition and high image quality, and if the image acquisition speed is increased, then SNR will suffer. [7, 10] OCT scanners laterally sample a target by steering the beam across one or two dimensions in order to produce a 2D image or a 3D volume. Processing the samples from the target to create an image is also a computationally intensive task, and the total time it takes to process the samples into an image can be higher than the line scan acquisition rate. There have been approaches to quickly process interferometer data into image volumes, and to render the analyzed OCT volumes at speeds suitable for real-time visualization, but for the most part, volumetric rendering still happens only post-process. In particular, attempts have been made to utilize Graphics Processing Units (GPUs) and Field-Programmable Gate Arrays (FPGAs) in order to improve the data processing and rendering. [15-22] Parallel programming approaches have also been followed to improve very high speed acquisition of OCT data, hide the data processing latency, and render 3D OCT volumes at real-time frame rates. [4, 20]

The focus of this paper is on a computationally simple image analysis algorithm that makes use of a Compute Unified Device Architecture (CUDA) enabled NVIDIA Quadro-5000 Graphics Processor Unit (GPU), which allows fast processing of 2D images to occur in real-time. Our algorithm will be integrated into a custom-built prototype SDOCT corneal imaging system that can scan 128,000 lines per second (128 kHz A-scan rate) with acceptable image quality (12-bits/pixel frequency sampling). Our implementation is tolerant of the low SNR in the images inherent with the necessarily short exposure times of the SDOCT spectrometer's line-scan camera. The algorithm (diagrammed in Fig. 1) automatically detects the shallowest surface of an imaged structure in 1.4-3.2 milliseconds, depending on the dimensions of the image (as discussed later), and hence has real–time applications. The algorithm will be incorporated into our existing augmented-reality SDOCT system for intra-operative surgical guidance. [23] In the future, the detected first tissue surface layer will be rendered in OpenGL, and then overlaid within the surgical microscope viewing environment, so as to appear in-situ within the actual corneal structure to provide real-time 3D visualization and surgical guidance for clinicians.

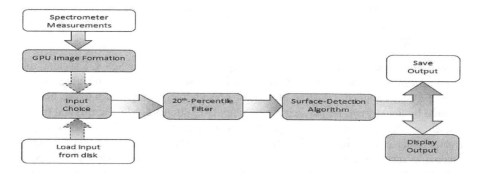

Fig. 1. A block diagram portraying the different stages in the algorithm. The CPU stages are shown in white blocks, while the GPU stages are shown in shaded blocks.

2 Methods

2.1 Prototype System Configuration

The prototype OCT system consists of an 840nm super luminescent diode (SLD) light source with 50nm bandwidth that feeds light into a broadband, single-mode fiber-optic Michelson Interferometer that splits the light into *sample-arm* and *reference-arm* sections. The sample-arm section interrogates the target sample being imaged. For this paper, the target sample was a static phantom model consisting of a piece of folded scotch tape embedded inside clear candle wax gel. Fig 2(a) shows a zoomed image of the phantom (with the embedded scotch-tape) as reconstructed by our OCT system. The reference-arm section physically matches the path length of the light traveling through the sample-arm section from the SLD source to the beginning of the target range in the sample. The light output from the sample arm and reference arm are combined back together in the interferometer, and fed into a spectrometer that measures the amplitudes of the individual frequency components of the received signal. The detected signal is processed into an A-scan 1D image, which is a depth profile of the various reflections of light from the distinct structural layers present in the sample. The A-scan represents a reflectivity profile along the beam for a fixed lateral scanning position of the scanning mechanism, and at a single fixed location on the target sample. Multiple A-scans are collected to form a 2D cross-sectional image of the target sample region being imaged. [24] The prototype SDOCT system has a scan depth range of 6mm, and acquires A-scans at 128 kHz when scanning 15 volumes per second resulting in lower contrast, lower quality SDOCT images than typical SDOCT systems. We do this to satisfy the physical space requirements for real-time surgical guidance. The SLD source has a total light output of ~6.76 mW, but the light output progressively decreases as it passes through the fibers and components in the SDOCT system. The power at the output of the sample-arm is 2.851 mW. The light returned by the sample is combined with the light output from the reference-arm in the interferometer, which filters out the light scattered in the sample, preserving only the small percentage of light that directly interrogated the subsurface targets for analysis by the spectrometer, where the input power is on the order of 50-100 nW.

2.2   Image Analysis

Noise Reduction. As a result of the rapid acquisition time of our SDOCT system, the output images are affected by substantial speckle noise. Since the manufacturer of our SDOCT system applied a custom non-linear noise reduction algorithm to the images acquired by the system, we chose not to attempt to explicitly model the residual noise. Instead, we chose to implement a post-processing algorithm that is insensitive to the remaining noise in the images. The integration time for all the frequency signals at the detector is very short, < 8 ns, and this contributes to the noise. SDOCT SNR also inherently drops off with depth, of particular relevance to our system with its extra deep 6mm A-scan length. Since the SNR depends in part on the light output power being detected at the spectrometer and the detector sensitivity, it follows that a generated image will have more noise and less contrast if the detected light output at the spectrometer is low. [24] Consequently, due to the noisy background, the physical edge boundaries are difficult to discriminate in the images generated by our SDOCT system.

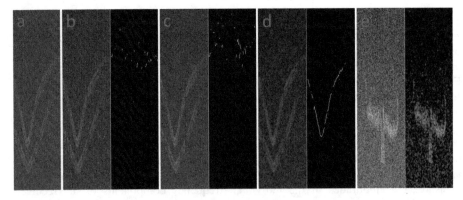

Fig. 2. (a) A zoomed view of an original noisy OCT image (b) Zoomed view of a bilateral filtered image (left), and the detected surface (right), (c) Zoomed view of a median filtered image (left), and the detected surface (right), (d) Zoomed view of a 20th-percentile and Gaussian filtered image (left), and subsequent detected surface (right), (e) Zoomed view of an extremely noisy OCT image (left), and the 20th-percentile and Gaussian filtered output (right), which resulted in significant noise reduction

Sufficiently fast conventional noise-reduction methods such as Gaussian blurring, or non-iterative edge-preserving smoothing methods such as Bilateral filtering, were unable to satisfactorily suppress the noise in the OCT images without substantial loss of contrast on the actual structures being scanned. When the surface detection algorithm (described next) was applied after bilateral filtering our test image, the detected shallow surface was false as shown in Fig 2 (b). Median filtering is one of the slowest non-iterative noise-reduction algorithms [25], and it is often used to remove speckle noise, but it also struggled with the large amplitude of the image noise, as shown in Fig 2 (c). A key insight into our problem is that while the background contains many pixels that are very bright due to noise, with several background patches containing over 50% bright noise pixels, these pixels are generally randomly scattered and intermixed with dark pixels. Only actual surfaces contain a *large* majority of bright pixels. Sharpening our images using a Laplacian filter (after smoothing using a Gaussian) did not improve our detection, albeit the contrast of the image improved. Since Laplacian filters approximate the second-order derivatives of the image [26], application of a Laplacian filter to the original image increased the noise by enhancing the intensity values of the noisy pixels in the background patches. So, a filter was required that would increase the edge contrast for any input image while darkening pixels that are not mostly surrounded by bright edge pixels. Percentile filers, also known as rank filters, are certainly not new to image processing, but aside from the Median filter, other percentile filters are typically not used directly for noise reduction or image restoration, but rather for more specialized tasks, such as estimating the statistical properties of image noise, surface relief etc. [27, 28, 29]

We believe that we are the first to apply non-median percentile filtering to OCT noise reduction, as well as to implement percentile filtering (for any purpose) on a GPU. For our particular OCT images, selecting 20th-percentile (first quintile) seemed to best suppress the noise while simultaneously increasing the contrast of the first surface in all of our images. The intensity of most pixels is adjusted by the percentile filter toward the dark end of the gray-level range, except for those pixels surrounded almost exclusively ($\geq 80\%$ of their neighbors) by bright pixels. The 20th percentile was calculated by first determining the ordinal rank n described by:

$$n = \left(\frac{P}{100} \times N\right) + \frac{1}{2} \tag{1}$$

where P is percentile that is required to be calculated (in our case $P = 20$), and N is the number of elements in the sorted array. A small 3×3 neighborhood was considered and so, $N = 9$. Substituting the above values in the formula yielded a rank of 2.3, and this value was then rounded to the nearest integer (i.e., 2). Next, the element in the sorted array that corresponds to rank 2 was taken to be the 20th percentile. Thus, for each pixel in the image, a sorted array containing nine elements corresponding to a 3×3 neighborhood around that pixel was extracted, and the second element in that sorted array was set as that pixel's intensity value. Small-neighborhood percentile filtering often leaves small-amplitude residual noise, and so we Gaussian blurred the image (with a 3×3 kernel) following the percentile filtering. Through this approach, the bright regions and edges were preserved, and noise was reduced in the image. Results of applying the 20th-Percentile filter and subsequent Gaussian blurring to various test images can be seen in Figs 2 (d) and (e), and Fig 3.

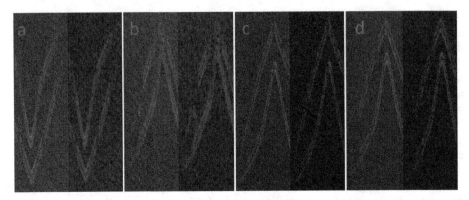

Fig. 3. Application of the 20th-percentile and Gaussian filters to four different OCT images. In (a), (b), (c), and (d), images on the left represent the zoomed views of the original noisy OCT images, while images on the right represent the corresponding zoomed views of the filtered images.

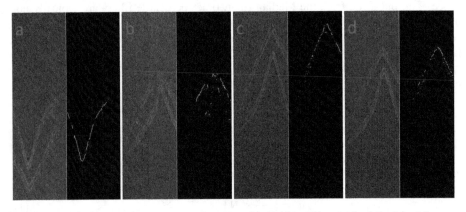

Fig. 4. Results of the surface-detection algorithm. In (a), (b), (c), and (d), the original images are shown on the left while the detected surfaces are shown on the right.

Detection of Surfaces. The goal of our preprocessing is to enable very fast surface-detection for robust, real-time operation. After the input OCT image is 20th-percentile and Gaussian filtered, an Otsu threshold for the entire grayscale OCT image is computed using Otsu's method. [30,31] Otsu's original filter uses a bimodal histogram containing two peaks, which represent the foreground and the background, to model the original grayscale image. The filter then tries to find an optimal threshold that separates the two peaks so that the variance within each region is minimal. If there are L gray-levels in the OCT image [1, 2, 3.... L], then the *within-class variance* is calculated for each gray level. The within-class variance is defined as the sum of weighted variances of the two classes of pixels (foreground and background), and it is represented by:

$$\sigma_w^2(t) = w_1(t)\sigma_1^2(t) + w_2(t)\sigma_2^2(t) \qquad (2)$$

where σ_w^2 is the within-class variance, σ_i^2 is the variance of a single (foreground or background) class, and w_i is the weight that represents the probabilities of the two classes separated by the threshold t. The gray level value for which the sum of weighted variances is lowest is set as the Otsu threshold. This approach is computationally intensive as it involves an exhaustive search for the threshold among all the gray-levels present in the 8-bit grayscale OCT image. A faster approach to threshold selection, also described by Otsu, involves the computation of the *between-class variance*. Otsu showed that maximizing the between-class variance led to the same result as minimizing the within-class variance [29, 30], and the between-class variance is given by:

$$\sigma_B^2(t) = \sigma_T^2(t) - \sigma_w^2(t) = w_1(t)w_2(t)[\mu_1(t) - \mu_2(t)]^2 \qquad (3)$$

where σ_B^2 is the between-class variance, σ_T^2 is the total variance of both classes, w_i are the class probabilities, and μ_i are the class means respectively. σ_B^2 and σ_w^2 are functions of the threshold, while σ_T^2 is not.

The class probability $w_1(t)$ is represented as a function of the threshold t by:

$$w_1(t) = \sum_0^t p_i \qquad (4)$$

where p_i is the probability distribution, which was obtained by normalizing the gray-level histogram, and the class mean $\mu_1(t)$ is calculated by:

$$\mu_1(t) = [\sum_0^t p(i) x(i)]/w_1 \qquad (5)$$

where $x(i)$ is the center of the ith histogram bin. Similarly, by using the same formulas above, $w_2(t)$ and $\mu_2(t)$ can be computed from the histogram for bins which are greater than t. The between-class variance calculation is a much faster and simpler approach to selecting a threshold that separates the foreground pixels from background pixels. Next, our surface detection algorithm performs a very efficient linear search along each individual column of the 20th-percentile filtered image for the first faintly visible surface. As the search iterates down each column (A-scan) in the preprocessed image, the algorithm compares each pixel's intensity value with its neighbors, and based upon the computed Otsu threshold, it determines if the current pixel is present in the background or the foreground of the image. By efficiently utilizing the pre-determined Otsu threshold, the surface-detection algorithm correctly selects the first surface for the majority of the columns in the image. These individual selected pixel localizations (one per column) are then pruned of outliers (as described below), and connected together into one or more curved sections, each of which corresponds to an unambiguous physically continuous segment of the underlying surface.

Isolated single-pixel outliers were easily removed, but small clusters of connected outliers were more challenging to remove in real-time. Fortunately, these clusters tended to be physically separated from the actual surface of interest, and so, they could be implicitly excluded during the curve-connecting stage. Detected pixels were connected together so as to find only the surface of interest by first measuring the distance between each set of two detected points, and then connecting them together by a rendered line. Sets of two points whose distance exceeded a given threshold were also connected together, but by a line of lower intensity, so that while the entire surface is automatically detected, there is also a visual cue to locations where ambiguity in the OCT image could possibly indicate that a small gap might be present in the physical tissue surface.

Table 1. Performance of the algorithm measured for five images

Image Number	Dimension	GPU execution time – 20th-Percentile Filter (milliseconds)	GPU execution time – Surface Detection (milliseconds)	CPU Execution Time – Surface Detection (milliseconds)
1	256 x 1024	~0.368	1.222	109
2	256 x 1024	~0.368	1.218	93
3	256 x 1024	~0.368	1.040	141
4	256 x 2048	~0.727	2.475	172
5	256 x 2048	~0.727	2.472	202
Average Execution Time (milliseconds)		~0.512	1.685	143.5

3   Results

The 20th-percentile filter, followed by Gaussian blurring, reduced large amounts of speckle noise in the image, which allowed the surface detection algorithm to quickly and accurately detect the shallowest surface present in the image. The surfaces detected by the algorithm for different images are shown in Fig 4, and the measured time it took to execute the entire algorithm on the GPU is shown in Table 1. The dimensions of B-scan OCT images that were passed as an input to the algorithm were varied, and this was intentionally done in order to measure the performance of the algorithm under this condition. On an average, the 20th-percentile filter implemented using CUDA on the GPU took ~0.512 milliseconds to execute. The detection of the surface from the 20th-percentile and Gaussian filtered image took ~1.7 milliseconds on average.

The surface-detection algorithm was also implemented on the CPU, and its performance was measured and found to be 143.5 milliseconds, on average. The original image and the detected curve's mask were overlaid using ITK-SNAP [32] as seen in Fig 5. From the overlaid images, it is visually noticeable that most of the detected surfaces match with the curved structures in the original image, with the total computation time being less than 3.5 milliseconds. However, the algorithm is not perfect, and the noise present in the original low-contrast OCT images does occasionally result in fractured surface detection as shown in Figs 5 and 6. The performance of the algorithm was timed using NVIDIA's Visual Profiler v4.2 and NVIDIA's Nsight Visual Studio Edition v3.2. On average, the total runtime of the program was 1.126 seconds, which included the low-bandwidth memory copies to and from the CPU and GPU. [33]

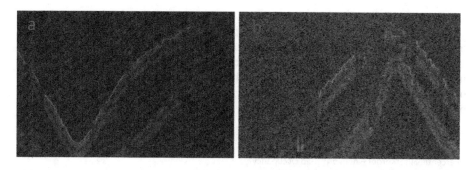

Fig. 5. Zoomed results showing two different original images with overlaid surface detection. In (a) and (b), the detected curve (shown in red) for each test image was overlaid on the original image. By visual inspection, the detected curves line up well with the original edges.

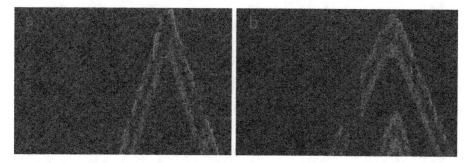

Fig. 6. Zoomed crops of the overlays for two different images in (a) and (b) show how a lack of differentiation in intensity between pixels representing an edge versus the background can cause the surface detection to be fractured by gaps

4   Discussion and Future Directions

The dimensions of the image play a vital role in the performance of the percentile filter. For a 256x1024 pixel image, the execution times were measured for the *PercentileFilterKernel* and *SurfaceDetectionKernel* on the GPU; the filtering stage took ~369μs to filter the image, while the surface-detection stage took 1.22ms to execute. Unlike a CPU that is optimized to handle sequential code that is complex and branching, a GPU is optimized for the parallel application of one piece of code (a *kernel*) to many elements at once (e.g., to each pixel in an image). With a GPU, each pixel's intensity value in the output image can be calculated by a dedicated thread, which is assigned to work on the corresponding pixel and its neighbors in the input image. As with a CPU, a GPU's fastest memory is its on-chip *registers* and its slowest memory is the bulk *global* GPU memory. Also, just like a CPU can speed global memory access by using a cache (for example: L1 cache), a GPU can speed access to its global memory by allocating a dedicated high-speed *shared* memory to each *block* of threads. During runtime, a block of threads executed by a streaming multiprocessor (SM) on the GPU is further grouped into *warps*, where a warp is a group of 32 parallel threads. The use of shared memory allows global memory access to be coalesced by warps, and thereby improves the latency of the data fetches. As shared memory is present on-chip, it has a latency that is roughly 100x lower than uncached global memory access, and it is allocated per block, which allows all parallel threads in a block to have access to the same high-speed shared memory. [33] GPUs also permit traditional L1 caching of memory, but the GPU L1 cache still has inferior performance to per-block shared memory in terms of memory bandwidth. [34]

PercentileFilterKernel – Active Thread Occupancy

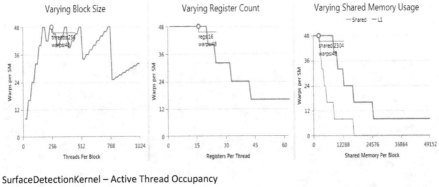

SurfaceDetectionKernel – Active Thread Occupancy

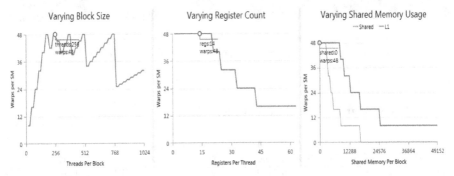

Fig. 7. Graphs detailing the current active thread occupancy on the GPU for the *PercentileFilterKernel* and *SurfaceDetectionKernel* respectively. The red circle shows the algorithm's active thread occupancy on the GPU as set against other theoretically calculated occupancy levels by NVIDIA's Nsight Visual Studio Edition v3.2.

The active thread occupancy levels for our algorithm are displayed in Fig 7, and the red circle in each graph represents the runtime state of the GPU as dictated by our algorithm. Occupancy can be measured in terms of warps, and it is defined as the ratio of the current number of active warps running concurrently on a streaming multiprocessor (SM) to the maximum number of warps that can run concurrently. [33] For the *PercentileFilterKernel*, there are 48 warps active on our GPU with the maximum number of warps for our GPU being 48. Thus, the occupancy level for the

Percentile Filter is 100%. From the graph detailing the varying block size for the *PercentileFilterKernel*, allocating 256 threads per block allowed an efficient coalesced global memory access. Out of these 256 threads per block, only 128 threads were used to load the neighbors of consecutive pixels to the shared memory. Each of these 128 threads processed a 3×3 or 5×5 neighborhood as set by the user, and loaded them into shared memory. The remaining 128 threads in the same block would access the "shared" pixels that were previously loaded by the first set of 128 threads, thus effectively reducing the read operation by half, and at the same time, creating a very efficient memory access pattern. In the two Fig 7 graphs titled "Varied Shared Memory Usage", the legend "L1" represents the cache memory present on the GPU, while the legend "Shared" represents the shared memory present on the GPU, as previously discussed. From the shared memory usage graph for the *PercentileFilterKernel*, it can be seen that the utilization of the shared memory on the GPU allows faster data access when compared to L1-cache memory of the GPU. Similarly, from the graphs for the *SurfaceDetectionKernel*, the occupancy was calculated to be 100%, with registers being sufficient so-as to not require or benefit from shared memory, and the active warp count equals the maximum number of warps running in parallel on the GPU. As seen from the varying block size graph for the *SurfaceDetectionKernel*, only 256 threads were used to detect the faintly visible surface. Each thread was allowed to process pixels only along a single column of the image. The thread extracted the values of the neighbors of a pixel, either in a 3×3 or 5×5 neighborhood as set by the user, loaded the values to memory, and used the computed Otsu threshold to determine if the pixel is present on the edge representing the phantom's surface.

However, the percentile filtering stage of the algorithm can be further optimized. In future work, the sorting scheme employed by the 20th-percentile filter could be upgraded in order to boost the performance of the algorithm. Presently, a naïve bubble sorting implementation is used by the algorithm. A naïve bubble sort is efficient in cases where only a 3×3 or a 5×5 pixel neighborhood is being considered, and only half the elements stored in the sorting array are being sorted, leading to a runtime of $O(n^2/4)$. However, as the size of the sorting array increases with neighborhood size, it becomes more efficient to run other sorting algorithms, such as radix sort or quick sort. [35, 36] Moving beyond the detection of the first surface, detecting underlying surfaces poses a challenge because these surfaces do not always appear smoothly connected or visible in the image. There may be gaps in the image that actually represent a structure in the target tissue being imaged, and it is important to represent these gaps by appropriate marker(s) in the image. Future directions of this algorithm are directed towards detecting and analyzing these underlying surfaces robustly, even when physical discontinuities are occasionally present.

5   Conclusion

We have implemented a GPU-based algorithm capable of real-time detection of first surfaces in noisy SDOCT images, such as those acquired by our prototype SDOCT corneal imaging system that trades off an inherently lower SNR for high-speed acquisition of images spanning 6mm in depth. The algorithm requires ~0.5 milliseconds on average to percentile and Gaussian filter the image, and ~1.7 milliseconds on average to detect the first surface thereafter. The surface detection algorithm's accuracy significantly depends on our preprocessing to reduce the speckle noise in the original image. More than 90% of the detected surface lies on the actual edge boundary. We are now incorporating our algorithm into a complete system for real-time corneal OCT image analysis and surgical guidance. Our implementation will enable clinicians to have an augmented-reality in-situ view of otherwise invisible tissue structures and surfaces during microsurgery.

Acknowledgements. This work was funded in part by NIH grants #R01EY021641 and #R21-EB007721, a grant from Research to Prevent Blindness, and a NSF graduate student fellowship.

References

1. LaRocca, F., Izzat, J.: Handheld simultaneous scanning laser ophthalmoscopy and optical coherence tomography system. Biomed. Opt. Express. 4, 2307–2321 (2013)
2. Fang, L., Izzat, J.: Fast Acquisition and Reconstruction of Optical Coherence Tomography Images via Sparse Representation. IEEE Trans. Act. Med. Imaging 32, 2034–2049 (2013)
3. Drexler, W., Fujimoto, J.G.: State-of-the-art retinal optical coherence tomography. Progr. Retinal Eye Res. 27, 45–88 (2008)
4. Jian, Y., Sarunic, M.: Graphics processing unit accelerated optical coherence tomography processing at megahertz axial scan rate and high resolution video rate volumetric rendering. J. Biomed. Opt. 18, 026002–026002 (2013)
5. An, L.: High speed spectral domain optical coherence tomography for retinal imaging at 500,000 A-lines per second. Biomed. Opt. Express. 2, 2770–2783 (2011)
6. Ricco, S., Chen, M., Ishikawa, H., Wollstein, G., Schuman, J.: Correcting motion artifacts in retinal spectral domain optical coherence tomography via image registration. In: Yang, G.-Z., Hawkes, D., Rueckert, D., Noble, A., Taylor, C. (eds.) MICCAI 2009, Part I. LNCS, vol. 5761, pp. 100–107. Springer, Heidelberg (2009)
7. Robinson, M.D., Izatt, J., Farsiu, S.: Novel applications of super-resolution in medical imaging. In: Milanfar, P. (ed.) Super-resolution Imaging, pp. 383–412. CRC Press (2010)
8. Tao, Y., Izzat, J.: Intraoperative spectral domain optical coherence tomography for vitreoretinal surgery. Opt. Lett. 35, 3315–3317 (2010)
9. Geerling, G.: Intraoperative 2-Dimensional Optical Coherence Tomography as a New Tool for Anterior Segment Surgery. Arch. Ophthalmol. 123, 253–257 (2005)
10. McNabb, R.P., Farsiu, S., Izatt, J.: Distributed scanning volumetric SDOCT formotion corrected corneal biometry. Biomed. Opt. Exp. 3, 2050–2065 (2012)
11. Gargesha, M., Jenkins, M.W., Rollins, A.M., Wilson, D.L.: Denoising and 4D visualization of images. Opt. Exp 16, 12313–12333 (2008)
12. Jian, Z., Yu, L., Rao, B., Chen, Z.: Three-dimensional speckle suppression in optical coherence tomography based on the curvelet transform. Opt. Exp 18, 1024–1032 (2010)
13. Wong, A., Mishra, A., Bizheva, K., Clausi, D.A.: General Bayesian estimation for speckle noise reduction in optical coherence tomography retinal imagery. Opt. Exp. 18, 8338–8352 (2010)
14. Salinas, H.M., Fernández, D.C.: Comparison of PDE-based nonlinear diffusion approaches for image enhancement and denoising in optical coherence tomography. IEEE Trans. Med. Imag. 26, 761–771 (2007)

15. Lee, K.K.C.: Real-time speckle variance swept-source optical coherence tomography using a graphics processing unit. Biomed. Opt. Express. 3, 1557–1564 (2012)
16. Li, J., Bloch, P.: Performance and scalability of Fourier domain optical coherence tomography acceleration using graphics processing units. Appl. Opt. 50, 1832–1838 (2011)
17. Rasakanthan, J., Sugden, K., Tomlins, P.H.: Processing and rendering of Fourier domain optical coherence tomography images at a line rate over 524 kHz using a graphics processing unit. J. Biomed. Opt. 16, 020505 (2011)
18. Sylwestrzak, M.: Real-time massively parallel processing of spectral optical coherence tomography data on graphics processing units. In: Proceedings of SPIE -Optical Coherence Tomography and Coherence Techniques, vol. 8091 (2011)
19. Watanabe, Y., Itagaki, T.: Real-time display on Fourier domainoptical coherence tomography system using a graphics processing unit. J. Biomed. Opt. 14, 060506 (2009)
20. Zhang, K., Kang, J.U.: Graphics processing unit-based ultrahigh speed real-time Fourier domain optical coherence tomography. IEEE J. Sel. Topics Quantum Electron. 18, 1270–1279 (2012)
21. Desjardins, A.E.: Real-time FPGA processing for high-speed optical frequency domain imaging. IEEE Trans. Med. Imag. 28, 1468–1472 (2009)
22. Ustun, T.E.: Real-time processing for Fourier domain optical coherence tomography using a field programmable gate array. Rev. Sci. Instrum. 79, 114301 (2008)
23. Galeotti, J., Schuman, J., Siegel, M., Wu, B., Klatzky, R., Stetten, G.: The OCT-Penlight: In-Situ Image Display for Guiding Microsurgery using OpticalCoherence Tomography (OCT). In: SPIE Medical Imaging, p. 7625-1 (2010)
24. Izatt, J.A., Choma, M.A.: Theory of Optical Coherence Tomography. In: Optical Coherence Tomography: Technology and Applications, Part 1, pp. 47–72 (2008)
25. Huang, T., Yang, G., Tang, G.: A fast two-dimensional median filtering algorithm. IEEE Trans. Acoust. Speech. Signal Process. 27, 13–18 (1979)
26. Shapiro, L., Stockman, G.: Computer Vision. Prentice Hall (2001)
27. Colom, M., Buades, A.: Analysis and Extension of the Percentile Method, Estimating a Noise Curve from a Single Image. Image Proc. On Line. 3, 332–359 (2013)
28. Percentile Filter, http://www.uoguelph.ca/~hydrogeo/Whitebox/Help/FilterPercentile.html
29. Percentile, Wikipedia, http://en.wikipedia.org/wiki/Percentile
30. Otsu, N.: A threshold selection method from gray-level histograms. IEEE Trans. Sys., Man., Cyber. 9, 62–66 (1979)
31. Otsu's Method, Wikipedia, http://en.wikipedia.org/wiki/Otsu's_method
32. Yushkevich, P., Piven, J., Gee, J., Gerig, G.: User-guided 3D active contour segmentation of anatomical structures: Significantly improved efficiency and reliability. Neuroimage 31, 1116–1128 (2006)
33. NVIDIA, CUDA C Best Practices Guide
34. NVIDIA, CUDA C Programming Guide
35. Sedgewick, R.: Algorithms in C++. Addison-Wesley (1998)
36. Sedgewick, R.: Implementing Quicksort Programs. Comm. ACM 21, 847–857 (1978)

Ultrasound Image Overlay onto Endoscopic Image by Fusing 2D-3D Tracking of Laparoscopic Ultrasound Probe

Ryo Oguma[1], Toshiya Nakaguchi[2], Ryoichi Nakamura[2], Tadashi Yamaguchi[2], Hiroshi Kawahira[2], and Hideaki Haneishi[2]

[1] Graduate School of Engineering, Chiba University
[2] Center for Frontier Medical Engineering, Chiba University
1-33 Yayoicho, Inage-ku, Chiba-shi, Chiba, 263-8522 Japan
r_oguma@chiba-u.jp

Abstract. In laparoscopic surgery, to identify the location of lesions and blood vessels inside organs, an ultrasound probe which can be inserted through small incision is used. However, since surgeons must observe the laparoscopic and ultrasound images both at the same time, it is difficult to understand the correspondence between the ultrasound image and real space. Therefore, to recognize the correspondence between these two images intuitively, we developed a system for overlaying ultrasound image on the laparoscopic image. Since the tip of the probe is flexed freely, we acquired the probe tip position and orientation using a method for detecting the probe angle from laparoscopic image and information obtained from optical tracking sensor. As a result of an experiment using a wire phantom, overlaying error of ultrasound images was found to be 0.97 mm. Furthermore, the rate of probe angle detection was evaluated through an animal experiment to be 83.1%.

1 Introduction

Since minimally invasive surgery is highly required for patients in modern medicine, these days, laparoscopic surgery is performed frequently. In laparoscopic hepatic surgery, to identify the location of lesions and blood vessels inside organs, an ultrasound (US) probe which can be inserted through small incision is used (LUS probe). However, since surgeons must observe the laparoscopic and US images both at the same time, it is difficult to understand the correspondence between the US image and real space. Therefore, to recognize the correspondence between these two images intuitively, augmented reality (AR) based surgical assistance such as overlaying US image on the laparoscopic image is carried out[1-3].

In order to overlay the US image correctly, the relative position of the LUS probe and laparoscope is required. To acquire the flexion angle of the probe tip, previous studies attempt to track it by attaching an electromagnetic (EM) tracking sensor on the tip[4,5]. There are also methods which detect a pattern attached on the probe tip by the laparoscope in order to obtain the pose and position of the tip without using any tracking sensors[6,7]. However, since it is necessary to capture a detailed pattern from

C.A. Linte et al. (Eds.): AE-CAI 2014, LNCS 8678, pp. 14–22, 2014.

laparoscopic image, the positional relationship between the probe and the laparoscope is limited. In addition, since it takes time for pattern detection, it may be difficult to overlay US image in real-time.

Therefore, we propose an optical and visual tracking method to calculate the LUS probe angle by detecting the probe tip from laparoscopic image. To detect the probe tip in laparoscopic image, we attached a thin color marker, which does not increase the diameter of the probe. Color marker detection of instrument in laparoscopic can be easily implemented in real-time, with high robustness[8]. Furthermore, optical tracking sensor is used in order to track the scope and instruments in AR surgery assistance[9-11]. Since the proposed system also uses only the optical tracking sensor, it has an advantage of the ability to combine with other computer-aided-surgery systems. For example, by attaching the optical marker to surgical instruments, it is possible to perform navigation, which presents the distance between the tip of the surgical instrument and the US image. Our study is about a system for real-time overlaying of US image onto laparoscopic image by detecting LUS probe angle flexion.

In this paper, we present the method of probe angle detection, accuracy evaluation of US image overlay, and the results of animal experiment.

2   System Overview

Fig.1 shows the flow of coordinate transformation and an overview of the system. The proposed system consists of three devices, a LUS probe (UST-5550 Hitachi-Aloka Medical Ltd.,Japan), a laparoscope and a position tracking sensor (MicronTracker 3, Sx60, Claron Technology Inc., Canada). We calculate the location of US image in the laparoscopic image coordinate system by tracking the positions of the LUS probe and laparoscope, where optical markers are attached at the handle, which is positioned outside the patient's body. We define the laparoscope marker as marker L and the LUS probe marker as marker P. Equation (1) denotes the transformation from X_U in the US image coordinate system to X_L in the laparoscope coordinate system.

$$X_L = T_{Lap}T_{LS}T_{SP}T_{US}X_U \qquad (1)$$

T_{LS} represents a transformation matrix from the optical sensor coordinate system to marker L coordinate system and T_{SP} represents a transformation matrix from marker P coordinate system to the optical sensor coordinates. These two matrices can be obtained from the output of the optical sensor when it detects the optical markers in real-time. T_{Lap} represents a transformation matrix from marker L coordinate system to the laparoscope coordinates. T_{US} represents a transformation matrix from US image coordinate system to marker P coordinate system.

T_{US} and T_{Lap} are needed for pre-operation calibration. T_{Lap} is obtained by using the corresponding points of the laparoscope coordinate system by camera calibration and the corresponding points of marker L coordinate system by optical sensor[12], while T_{US} changes depending on LUS probe angle. We will explain about LUS probe calibration in the next section.

3   LUS Probe Calibration

3.1   Probe Angle Detection

Fig.2 shows the LUS probe that we use. The probe tip has a rotational degree of free-dom of one axis, the angle $\angle ABC$ varies from $\pi / 3$ to $5\pi / 3$ rad by operating the wheel close at hand. Since only marker P is attached to the probe handle, the position of point A, which is inside the patient's body, cannot be estimated. Here, by obtaining the coordinates of the probe tip in the laparoscopic image, we have constructed a me-thod for detecting the probe angle. Fig.3 shows an overview of LUS probe angle de-tection method. First, we define the plane passing through the three points A, B and C of Fig.2. This plane is referred to as *flexion plane* in the rest of this paper. B and C were defined manually using a stylus. Position and orientation of the flexion plane is determined by the transformation matrix T_{SP} in Fig.1. Also this plane is parallel to the plane of marker P. Second, from the optical axis of the laparoscope, we find a vector extending to the probe tip of the laparoscopic image. By calculating the intersection of the flexion plane and the vector, the coordinates of A can be obtained, and we cal-culate the probe angle from three points, including B and C. In this study, we use green color markers for detection of the probe tip in the laparoscopic image, and detect the coordinate values in the image by image processing.

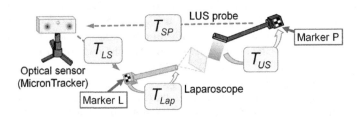

Fig. 1. Overview of the proposed system

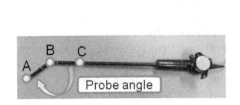

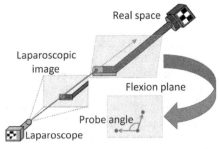

Fig. 2. Laparoscopic ultrasound probe, UST-5550

Fig. 3. Probe angle detection using laparoscopic image

3.2   Probe Calibration

After we detect the probe angle using the method mentioned above, we also need to acquire T_{US}. In this study, we prepared the conversion table from the probe angle to T_{US} with large numbers of their pairs. In order to obtain a large number of T_{US}, we have attached an additional marker to the probe tip for the optical tracking sensor. We define this marker as marker T. First, we calculate the transformation matrix T_{TU} to marker T coordinate system from the US image coordinates (Fig.4). We obtained T_{TU} using marker T and US image coordinate system of the corresponding points by wire phantom[13]. T_{TU} is constant regardless of probe angle.

Second, we find the transformation matrices T_{PT} to marker P from marker T coordinate system (Fig.5). From the position and orientation of marker T and P which are detected in each frame by freely changing the flexion angle of the probe tip, we continuously find sets of the probe angle and transformation matrix T_{PT}. Accordingly, we can obtain $T_{PT}(\theta)$ when the probe angle is θ. After obtaining the $T_{PT}(\theta)$ about 1000 sets, we would have created the conversion table.

Using T_{PT} and T_{TU}, we can now calculate transformation matrix T_{US}. We select the T_{PT} which is closest to the computed angle θ. Equation (2) shows the transformation matrix T_{US} when the probe angle is θ.

$$T_{US} = T_{PT}(\theta)T_{TU} \tag{2}$$

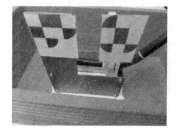 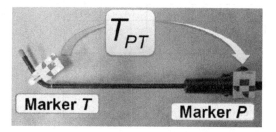

Fig. 4. Probe calibration of US image to marker T coordinate system

Fig. 5. LUS probe fitted with markers

4   Accuracy Evaluation of US Image Overlay

An accuracy evaluation was conducted by comparing feature points in laparoscopic image with points in US image. We used a normal camera (UCAM-DLF30, ELECOM Ltd., Japan, resolution 640 x 480 pixels) instead of laparoscope in this experiment setup. For the accuracy evaluation, we used a handmade phantom model shown in Fig.6, which consists of cross wire sets stretching between walls, where the intersections of cross wire is captured by the LUS. At the same time, the intersections are taken by the normal camera as shown in Fig.7. In consideration of relative position between the organ and laparoscope in surgery, this phantom is about 10~15cm away from the camera. We have taken 20 images by changing the position and orientation of the camera and probe angle. Fig.8 shows a camera image with overlaying semi-transparent US image by calculating the average of the original camera image and overlaid image. The feature points of the two sets is obtained for each image by manually selecting the wire intersections in camera image, and calculating the center point and the line segment. Then, high intensity points in overlaying US image is selected manually as two feature points, to calculate the center point and the line segment as well. Overlaying error is derived by Euclidean distance between the center point of the wire intersection and the center point of the feature points of US image, while rotation error is derived from the difference between the inclination of the line segment and scaling error is derived from the ratio of the length of the line segment. Calibration accuracy of the optical sensor is 0.25mm RMS[14], where calibration accuracy of the camera is 2.7mm RMS, which is the error between corresponding points used in the calculation of the transformation matrix T_{Lap} and re-projected points to the camera coordinate system using T_{Lap}. Calibration and re-projection was done 10 times, then the mean value was calculated.

Table 1 shows the results of the accuracy evaluation. The mean translation error was 0.97mm from the focal length of the camera. From this result, we found that the mean overlaying accuracy is amply high. However, the maximum error and standard deviation was large. The maximum value of translation error, rotation error, and scaling error was 4.3mm, 18.4 degrees, and 12.3%, respectively.

Table 1. Overlaying error. Mean, max, and standard deviation (SD) of 20 samples.

	Mean	Max	SD
Translation error(mm)	0.97	4.3	1.0
Rotation error(deg)	4.0	18.4	4.0
Scaling error(%)	4.4	12.3	3.7

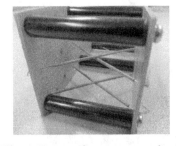

Fig. 6. Phantom for accuracy evaluation

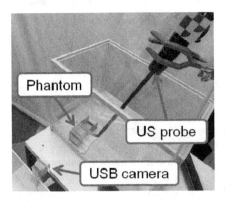

Fig. 7. Geometry of accuracy evaluation

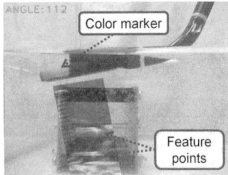

Fig. 8. Camera image overlaying US image

5   *In vivo* Evaluation

5.1   Clinical Feasibility Evaluation

The usability of the proposed system was assessed on animal experiment using a pig. In addition to the optical sensor and the LUS probe mentioned above, a PC (Windows 7, 32bit, Intel(R) Core(TM) i7-2600K CPU3.40GHz, RAM 4GB) and a laparoscope (IMAGE1 H3-Z, KARL STORZ, Germany, resolution 720 x 480 pixel) were used. An overview of the proposed system being used in animal experiments is shown in Fig. 9. All experiments were carried out laparoscopically. The probe which was inserted through 12mm diameter trocar is set onto the porcine liver. By tracking the marker mounted on the probe handle and the laparoscope, the system was carried out at 30fps overlaying in real-time. Since the sensor output is of 80 frames average, when the probe tip was moved, a delay of about 2 seconds occurred to move the US image overlaid position to the correct position. An overlaying image is shown in Fig. 10(a), and semi-transparent overlay image is shown in Fig. 10(b). The image of Fig. 10(a), since the opaque US image is overlapped directly over the laparoscopic image, understanding of the depth direction between images was difficult. In contrast, in the semi-transparent overlay image of Fig. 10(b), the intuitive recognition of the depth of vessel position was enhanced by the color of Doppler mode.

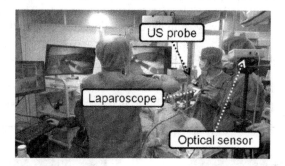

Fig. 9. Geometry of animal experiment

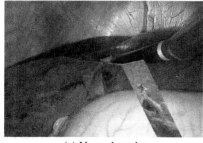
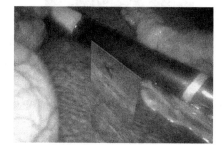

(a) Normal mode   (b) Semi-transparent mode

Fig. 10. US images are overlaid on laparoscopic image for the proposed system. The color regions on the US overlays represent blood flow inside an organ.

5.2   Angle Detection Rate Evaluation

When the color marker of the probe tip is detected from laparoscopic image, it is possible to calculate the probe angle to overlay the ultrasound image. Therefore, detection rate of the color marker was evaluated from the video sequence of laparoscope taken in the animal experiment. The percentage of the color marker in the shooting time (the time when the probe did not appear completely were excluded, e.g. during lens cleaning) was detected correctly. The pixel values in the laparoscopic image were converted from RGB to HSV color space, then we determined the following threshold condition to detect the color marker stably.

$$60 < H < 220, \quad S > 90, \quad V > 80 \tag{3}$$

Range of hue(H) is 0 to 360. Ranges of saturation(S) and value(V) are 0 to 255. After the thresholding, morphological opening processing was performed to remove noise. Fig.11(a) shows a laparoscopic image, and Fig.11(b) shows an extracted image given by the above process. Coordinates of the probe tip in the laparoscopic image was obtained by calculating the centroid of the high intensity pixels from Fig.11(b).

Table 2 shows the total recording time and results of the detection rate. The color marker detection rate was 83.1%, and the maximum continuous detection time was 241.9 seconds. In this experiment, false detection of the color marker did not occur. The maximum time of undetectable state was 42.1 seconds. This happens mainly when the probe tip is too far away from the camera, because of low illumination.

Table 2. Results of the color marker detection rate evaluation

Total time (s)	Detection success rate (%)	Maximum continuous detection time (s)	Maximum continuous non-detection time(s)
2009(33m29s)	83.1	241.9	42.1

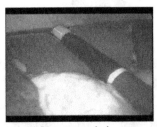

(a) Laparoscopic image   (b) Color marker detection image

Fig. 11. Results of the detection of the color marker from laparoscopic image

6   Discussion

Here we discuss about the experiments in Section 4 and Section 5, and the usefulness of surgical support system using the LUS probe angle detection.

The dispersion of overlaying precision causes error when the transformation matrices $T_{PT}(\theta)$ is calculated. The marker T and P shown in Fig.5 are used in this task, in order to put both markers into the measurement range of the optical sensor, it is necessary to keep a large distance between the probe and the optical sensor. It appears that as a result, when the measurement was performed near the border of the field of optical sensor's view, dispersion occurred. Although output average of the optical sensor is taken currently to address the dispersion issue, it is necessary to improve by using interpolation technique to remove outliers as the next task. Furthermore, a delay of about 2 seconds occurs in overlaying of the US image. Since LUS probe was not moved quickly during the operation, the influence of the delay was small. However when the overlaying image is observed while moving the laparoscope, this delay cannot be ignored. It is believed that by replacing the optical sensor with another sensor with wider range and higher accuracy, the output would be stabilized. Thus, improvement of the delay and dispersion of the overlaying precision is to be expected.

The proposed system is required to detect the color markers from the laparoscopic image and output of the optical sensor. Probe tip detection failed only when it is placed far from the laparoscope due to low illumination. The addition of computer vision techniques such as shape recognition, detection accuracy will be improved further. As mentioned in Section 1, since diameter of the probe tip does not increase even when the color marker is attached, means that it can be handled without a problem. It is also possible to carry out sterilization of the probe easily.

In this study, we developed a system for overlaying an ultrasound image on the laparoscopic image in real-time using probe angle detection. Future works consists of consideration of overlay representation method of the US image and improvement of calibration accuracy. In addition, we need to consider an algorithm to cope with multi-directional probe flex.

References

1. Peterhans, M., vom Berg, A., Dagon, B., et al.: A navigation system for open liver surgery: design, workflow and first clinical applications. The International Journal of Medical Robotics and Computer Assisted Surgery 7, 7–16 (2011)
2. Sindram, D., McKillop, I.H., Martinie, J.B., et al.: Novel 3-D laparoscopic magnetic ultrasound image guidance for lesion targeting. International Hepato-Pancreato-Biliary Association 12, 709–716 (2010)
3. Langø, T., Vijayan, S., Rethy, A., et al.: Navigated laparoscopic ultrasound in abdominal soft tissue surgery. technological overview and perspectives. International Journal of Computer Assisted Radiology and Surgery 7, 585–599 (2012)
4. Harms, J., Feussner, H., Baumgartner, M., et al.: Three-dimensional navigated laparoscopic ultrasonography. Surgical Endoscopy 15, 1459–1462 (2001)
5. Nakamoto, M., Nakada, K., Sato, Y., et al.: Intraoperative Magnetic Tracker Calibration Using a Magneto-Optic Hybrid Tracker for 3-D Ultrasound-Based Navigation in Laparoscopic Surgery. IEEE Trans. Medical Imaging 27, 255–270 (2008)
6. Edgcumbe, P., Nguan, C., Rohling, R.: Calibration and Stereo Tracking of a Laparoscopic Ultrasound Transducer for Augmented Reality in Surgery. In: Liao, H., Linte, C.A., Masamune, K., Peters, T.M., Zheng, G. (eds.) MIAR 2013 and AE-CAI 2013. LNCS, vol. 8090, pp. 258–267. Springer, Heidelberg (2013)

7. Jayarathne, U.L., McLeod, A.J., Peters, T.M., Chen, E.C.S.: Robust Intraoperative US Probe Tracking Using a Monocular Endoscopic Camera. In: Mori, K., Sakuma, I., Sato, Y., Barillot, C., Navab, N. (eds.) MICCAI 2013, Part III. LNCS, vol. 8151, pp. 363–370. Springer, Heidelberg (2013)
8. Bouarfa, L., Akman, O., Schneider, A., et al.: In-vivo real-time tracking of surgical instruments in endoscopic video. Minimally Invasive Therapy 21, 129–134 (2012)
9. Liao, H., Tsuzuki, M., Mochizuki, T., et al.: Fast image mapping of endoscopic image mosaics with three-dimensional ultrasound image for intrauterine fetal surgery. Minimally Invasive Therapy 18, 332–340 (2009)
10. Gavaghan, K.A., Peterhans, M., Oliveira-Santos, T., et al.: A Portable Image Overlay Projection Device for Computer-Aided Open Liver Surgery. IEEE Trans on Biomedical Engineering 58, 1855–1864 (2011)
11. Hansen, C., Wieferich, J., Riffer, F., et al.: Illustrative visualization of 3D planning models for augmented reality in liver surgery. International Journal of Computer Assisted Radiology and Surgery 5, 133–141 (2010)
12. Yamaguchi, T., Nakamoto, M., Sato, Y., et al.: Development of a camera model and calibration procedure for oblique-viewing endoscopes. Computer Aided Surgery 9(5), 203–214 (2004)
13. Chen, T.K., Thurston, A.D., Ellis, R.E., et al.: A Real-Time Freehand Ultrasound Calibration System with Automatic Accuracy Feedback and Control. Ultrasound in Medical & Biology 35, 79–93 (2009)
14. Claron Technology Inc.: MicronTracker 3, Specifications (2013),
    http://www.clarontech.com/microntracker-specifications.php

Simulation of Ultrasound Images
for Validation of MR to Ultrasound Registration
in Neurosurgery

Hassan Rivaz and D. Louis Collins

McConnell Brain Imaging Center
McGill University, Montreal, QC, Canada

Abstract. Image registration is an essential step in creating augmented environments and performing image-guided interventions. Registration algorithms are commonly validated against simulation and real data. Both validations are critical in a comprehensive analysis: On one hand, the simulation data provides ground truth registration results and can therefore accurately measure the performance of algorithms. It is also flexible and can include different levels of noise and outlier data. On the other hand, real data include factors that are not modeled in simulations and is therefore used to test algorithms against real-world applications. Simulated MR images are provided in the BrainWeb database and have been extensively used to validate and improve image registration algorithms. Simulated US images that correspond to these MR images are of great interest due to the growing interest in the use of ultrasound (US) as a real-time modality that can be easily used during interventions. In this work, we first generate digital brain phantoms by distribution of US scatterers based on the tissue probability maps provided in BrainWeb. We then generate US images of these digital phantoms using the publicly available Field II program. We show that these images look similar to the real US images of the brain. Furthermore, since both the US and MR images are simulated from the same tissue probability map, they are perfectly registered. We then deform the digital phantoms to simulate brain deformations that happen during neurosurgery, and generate US images of the deformed phantoms. We provide some examples for the use of such simulated US images for testing and enhancing image registration algorithms.

1 Introduction

An important step in generating augmented reality and image-guided operations is accurate alignment of different images of the tissue, such as magnetic resonance (MR) and ultrasound (US). Since the ground truth alignment between these images is rarely known in real tissue, validation of image registration algorithms is a challenging task. Open access databases that are used for validation include the Retrospective Image Registration Evaluation (RIRE) database [1], which contains MR, CT and positron emission tomography (PET) images of the brain,

C.A. Linte et al. (Eds.): AE-CAI 2014, LNCS 8678, pp. 23–32, 2014.

and Brain Images of Tumors for Evaluation (BITE) database [2], which provides ultrasound (US) and MR images. To allow validation of registration results, physical fiducials in RIRE or manually selected homologous anatomical landmarks in BITE can be used. While these databases test the algorithms against challenging real images, they have two limitations. First, the fiducial/landmark localization error limits the accuracy of the ground truth. Second, landmarks are limited to few points in the volumes and therefore registration accuracy throughout the volumes cannot be estimated.

Simulated images address these issues, and are usually included as (a necessary, but not sufficient) part of the validation experiments. As an example, the BrainWeb database [3] provides simulated T1-, T2- and proton-density- (PD-) weighted magnetic resonance (MR) images of the brain. The MR images are estimated from a probabilistic brain tissue type probability map. This database has been extensively used for validation of the image registration algorithms, evidenced by over 1200 citations [4].

Currently, no publicly available simulated dataset is available for testing and validating US registration algorithms. With the rapid growth of US in image-guided interventions and the need to register the intra-operative US (iUS) images to pre-operative acquisitions (commonly MR or CT), simulation of US images is of great importance.

In this work, we simulate realistic US images of brain using the Field II program [5]. Since US is generally used for imaging soft tissue, a deformable registration is needed to accurately register iUS to the pre-operative images in many image-guided surgical/radiotherapy applications. In this paper, we start from tissue probability maps provided in BrainWeb, generate digital US phantoms, and simulate 2D US images of the digital phantom from different orientations. We then deform the digital phantom to simulate brain deformation (i.e. brain shift), and generate US images of the deformed phantom. We generate US images from three simulated craniotomy locations of the brain with three different (zero, small and large) deformation levels. Outlier data is also commonly present in image registration problems; an example is the tumor resection area in the US image that does not correspond to the tumor in the MR image. To simulate the outlier data in US images, we change tissue probability maps at some regions, generating two US images with and without outliers at every location. Finally, at each craniotomy location, we simulate 100 2D US slices separated in the out-of-plane direction by 0.2 mm, similar to BITE database where the 2D handheld probe is swept on the tissue to generate 3D US. We will make this data publicly available.

US simulation is computationally expensive; simulation of a single US slice takes 9 hours on a 3 GHz CPU. Therefore, the total time for simulation of two sequence of 100 US slices corresponding to before and after compression of the phantom takes 75 days. We hope that making this data publicly available speeds testing and improving US registration algorithms.

This paper is organized as follows. In the next section, we elaborate the Field II simulation algorithm, construction of the digital US phantoms with and

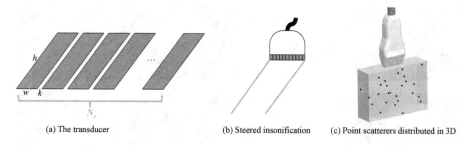

(a) The transducer   (b) Steered insonification   (c) Point scatterers distributed in 3D

Fig. 1. The transducer and digital phantom. (a) shows the zoomed transducer, consisting of N_e piezoelectric elements with height h, width w and kerf k. (b) shows the a steered insonification. Many such insonifications are performed in different angles to generate the fan-shaped image in phased array probes. (c) shows the digital phantom, where many US scatterers are distributed randomly. We place approximately 8 scatterers per cubic mm in our simulations as suggested by [5].

without outliers and deformation of the US phantoms. We then present the results, followed by conclusions and future work directions.

2   Methods

An ultrasound probe usually consists of many small piezoelectric elements that convert electric voltage to ultrasonic wave (Fig. 1 (a)). Each element is capable of both generating US waves using electric voltage, and listening for wave reflections from the tissue and converting acoustic signals to electrical voltage. To generate a typical 2D B-mode US image, a most basic strategy would be to generate one line from each element. However, some (or all) of the elements are excited together with pre-calculated time delay and amplitude to focus the beam at a desired location or to steer it in a desired direction (Fig. 1 (b)). Similarly, when the acoustic reflection is received in multiple elements, pre-specified delays and gains are used to average the signals. Transmit and receive focusing and steering are referred to as *beamforming* and significantly improve the quality of US images. We set all N_e elements in Field II simulations as active elements for beamforming to generate high quality images.

Each piezoelectric element at the US probe generates acoustic pressure in the form of a short sinusoidal pulse modulated with a Hanning or Gaussian window function. We use a Gaussian modulated excitation:

$$e(t) = \exp\left(-\frac{(t-\mu)^2}{2\sigma^2}\right) \cdot \sin(2\pi f_0 t) \tag{1}$$

where t is time, f_0 is the probe's center frequency, μ is the mean and σ^2 is the variance of the Gaussian function. Let $g(-\mathbf{x}, t)$ be the impulse response of the transducer, i.e. the pressure field generated from a Dirac delta excitation at the

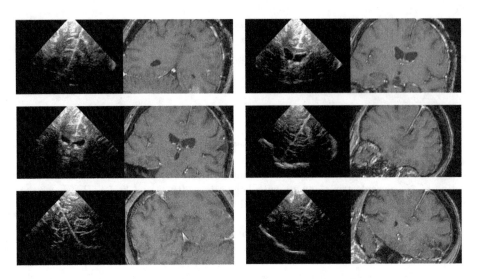

Fig. 2. Six examples of the intra-operative B-mode US and the corresponding pre-operative MR images from the BITE database. Note that the sulci and ventricles appear respectively hyperechoic and hypoechoic in the US images.

transducer at location $\mathbf{x}$ and time t. Field II performs the following convolution to calculate the radio-frequency (RF) data $r(\mathbf{x_0}, t)$ at a particular point $\mathbf{x_0}$ and time t [6,7]:

$$r(\mathbf{x_0}, t) = e(t) \underset{t}{*} g(-\mathbf{x}, t) \underset{\mathbf{x}}{*} s(\mathbf{x}) \Big|_{\mathbf{x}=\mathbf{x_0}} \tag{2}$$

where $\underset{t}{*}$ and $\underset{\mathbf{x}}{*}$ respectively denote temporal and spatial convolution, and s is the scattering medium. Field II allows placement of point scatterers with the desired scattering amplitude and location in the medium (e.g. Fig. 1 (c)). In the next section, we describe how we distribute scatterers in the brain phantom.

2.1 Scatterer Distribution

A portion of the US wave gets reflected when the acoustic impedance of the medium changes. Part of this reflection is because of microscopic changes in tissue properties, which is referred to as diffuse scattering. Another part is due to changes at the macroscopic level, e.g. at the boundary of gray matter (GM) and cerebrospinal fluid (CSF) (see [8] for more details). We incorporate both reflection sources in our digital brain phantom.

To model diffuse scattering, we spread many point scatterers (8 per cubic mm) throughout the phantom with normally distributed scattering amplitude. The scattering properties of white matter (WM), GM and CSF are different. Therefore, we follow previous work [9] that simulates US images from MRI. They suggest the intensity values of 32, 12 and 4 for respectively GM, WM and CSF,

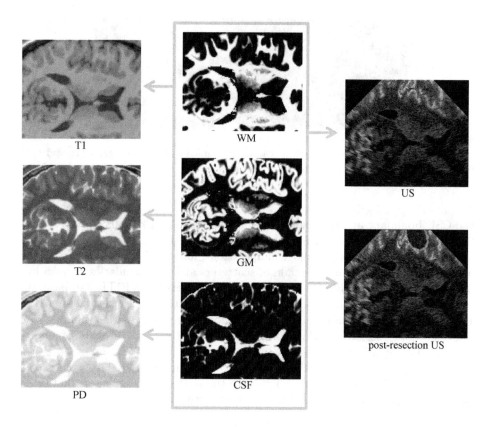

Fig. 3. Simulation of MR and US images from tissue probability maps in the middle column. Parts of the WM, GM and CSF are altered in the post-resection US image to simulate tissue resection.

and show that the simulated US images can be registered to real US images using cross correlation. Hence, we multiply the amplitude of scatterers intensity by these values based on their probabilistic tissue type determined by the BrainWeb phantom.

The ratio of US wave reflected at the boundary between two tissues with acoustic impedances Z_1 and Z_2 is $(Z_1 - Z_2)^2/(Z_1 + Z_2)^2 \cdot \cos(\theta)$, where θ is the incident angle. We calculate θ at every boundary by performing a dot product between the radial US wave and the normal of CSF tissue probability map edges[1]. Since acoustic impedance values for different brain tissue types are not available, we use the BITE database to approximate the reflection values. We therefore multiply scatterer intensities by the gradient magnitude of CSF tissue probability. The reflection at sulci CSF is significantly stronger compared to

---

[1] Since the boundary between WM and GM is not generally sharp, it is usually not visible under US. However, the boundary between CSF and WM or GM is sharp and is visible in US, and therefore we only consider CSF edges.

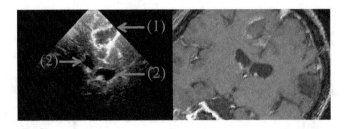

Fig. 4. Post-resection US and pre-operative MR images of neurosurgery. (1) and (2) respectively refer to the resection cavity and ventricles. The tumor region in MR does not correspond to the resection cavity in US.

the CSF boundary at the ventricle regions (see Fig. 2). Previous work [10] has in fact used this enhancement to perform US-MR registration. We therefore locate sulci area using morphological operations, followed by manual correction, and further multiply the amplitude of scatterers at CSF boundaries at sulci by 32. We select this number by investigating images from the BITE database. It should be noted that based on time gain control (TGC) and other factors, the US intensity at sulci can be different. Therefore, there is no perfect number for intensity values selected in this work. Fig. 3 shows the tissue probability maps and T1, T2 and PD weighted MR images from the BrainWeb, along with the simulated US image. Since both US and MR images are simulated from the same tissue probability map, they are aligned. In the next section, we alter the tissue probability maps to generate US images with outliers.

2.2   US Images with Outliers

Tumor resection and bleeding are among the sources of outliers when registering US and MR images of the BITE database. We simulate tumor resection by changing the WM, GM and CSF tissue types inside an elliptical region to a new hypoechoic type that contains weak scatterers. This is in accordance with real data where the resection region is filled with saline solution and diluted blood (i.e. a weak scattering mixture). We set the scatterer intensity in the resected region to 6 to simulate images that look similar to real images. Another source of artifact in the post-resection US images comes from Surgicel (Ethicon, Somerville, NJ), a surgical hemostat that is often used after resection to stop bleeding. Surgicel generates bright edges around the tumor as shown in Fig. 4. We model this edges in our simulations by placing scatterers around the resection cavity.

2.3   Deformation of the Simulated Phantoms

The brain tissue deforms after the craniotomy and during the surgery due to bio-chemical and physical factors. The deformation can be as much as 38 mm [11] in some areas. We deform the digital US phantom, by moving its scatterers, using free-form B-spline transformations. In real brain deformation, the maximum displacement of the brain happen around the cortex where craniotomy is performed. We therefore linearly decrease the deformation of the B-spline nodes from the cortex to achieve the deformation shown in Fig. 5 (b). Other deformations that use finite element simulation of viscoelastic tissue models are also possible. It should be noted that we deform the digital phantom (i.e. displace scatterers) and not the BrainWeb tissue probability maps. This is in accordance with reality, where the scatterers move with the brain as it deforms. We deform the digital phantom at two levels with maximum deformation levels of 5 mm and 40 mm.

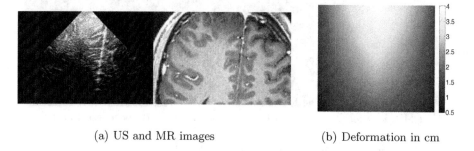

(a) US and MR images   (b) Deformation in cm

Fig. 5. The US and MR images in (a) are from the BITE database. The simulated deformation in (b) is the highest close to the cortex (top center), where brain shift is usually the largest.

2.4   Simulation Time

Simulation of a single US slice takes 9 hours on a 3 GHz CPU. Therefore, simulating 100 slices of a sweep takes 37 days. We simulate US slices in 3 locations with 3 different levels of compression (zero, small and large) with 2 different phantoms with and without the resection cavity. Therefore, the total computation time is $3 \times 3 \times 2 \times 37 = 675$ days. Providing this data online can help the

Table 1. Imaging and US probe parameters (see also Fig. 1)

symbol	description	value
w	width of elements	0.11 mm
h	height of elements	5 mm
k	kerf (dist. between elements)	0.011 mm
N_e	number of all elements	128
N_a	number of active elements	128
f_0	center frequency	7 MHz
f_s	sampling frequency	100 MHz
α	attenuation	35 dB/m
α_{f0}	attenuation center frequency	7 MHz
α_f	frequency dependent attenuation	5 dB/(MHz.m)

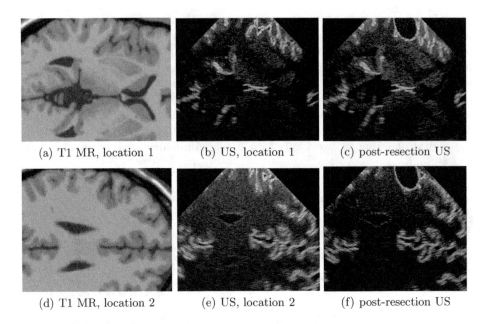

(a) T1 MR, location 1   (b) US, location 1   (c) post-resection US

(d) T1 MR, location 2   (e) US, location 2   (f) post-resection US

Fig. 6. The simulated US images at two different locations. The T1 images are from the BrainWeb. The post-resection US images simulate tumor resection and contain outlier data.

academic and industrial research groups in testing and validating novel image registration algorithms.

3   Results

The size of the piezoelectric elements and their distance (Fig. 1) are confidential manufacturer information. We therefore use the values provided in Field II: $w = 0.11$ mm, $h = 5$ mm, $k = 0.011$ mm and $N_e = 128$ (see Fig. 1). We also set the probe's center frequency f_0 to 7 MHz, the sampling frequency f_s to 100 MHz, the focal point of transmitted wave to half of the image depth, and use all $N_e = 128$ elements for transmit and receive beamforming. The value of these parameters are summarized in Table 1.

Field II generates RF data, which is not suitable for visualization because it is modulated with a high frequency ($f_0 = 7$ MHz) carrier (see [12] for more details). Therefore, we calculate the envelope of the RF signal and perform a log compression of the resulting amplitudes to reduce the dynamic range of the envelope. The resulting image is similar to what is commonly seen as a B-mode image on a US scanner. We have simulated US images from three different locations of the brain. Fig. 6 shows the simulated US images, along with BrainWeb T1 MR images, at two locations (the third location is shown in Fig. 3).

The digital phantom is in 3D, and we simulate series of 2D US images that sweep the 3D phantom, similar to the BITE database. The sweeps of 2D US images can then be simply stacked together to generate 3D US volumes.

4   Discussion

Simulated US images can be used to test and validate numerous kinds of image analysis algorithms. First, the deformed US volume and the T1 (or T2 or PD) MR volume can be used to test 3D volumetric registration algorithms. Second, the individual US images and the T1 (or T2 or PD) MR volume can be used to test 2D-3D (i.e. slice to volume) registration algorithms. Third, the post-resection US images and the MR volume can be used to test the robustness of registration algorithms to outlier data. Forth, the US images with and without deformation can be used to test US-US registration algorithms. Fifth, the US images with the small deformation magnitude, the US images with the large deformation magnitude and the MR images can be used to test group-wise registration algorithms, where all three volumes are considered simultaneously to improve the accuracy and robustness of registration algorithm.

The deformation model using the free-form B-splines is purely geometrical and does not respect the mechanical properties of the brain. For example, the deformation of the fluid CSF is fundamentally different from that of WM and GM. Finite element analysis has been used in the past to generate deformation fields that take into account tissue mechanical properties [13,14]. Similar analysis can be used to generate more realistic brain shift deformation maps.

The intensity of B-mode image in different regions of the brain are provided in [9], which we used to set the scatterer amplitudes. However, the relationship between the scatterer intensity and B-mode intensity is rather complex and subject of research [15,16,7]. Nevertheless, these values produced simulated images that are visually similar to the real images from the BITE database. Rigorous validation of the simulated images is a subject of future work.

5   Conclusions

Validation is a critical and challenging step in the development of novel image registration algorithms. In this work, we showed how realistic US images can be simulated from tissue probability maps of the BrainWeb database. Along with the BrainWeb database that provides MR images with different noise and intensity non-uniformity levels, the simulated US images can be used to test and improve various types of image registration algorithms.

References

1. West, J., Fitzpatrick, J.M., Wang, M.Y., Dawant, B.M., Maurer Jr., C.R., Kessler, R.M., Maciunas, R.J., Barillot, C., Lemoine, D., Collignon, A., et al.: Comparison and evaluation of retrospective intermodality brain image registration techniques. Journal of Computer Assisted Tomography 21, 554–568 (1997)

2. Mercier, L., Del Maestro, R.F., Petrecca, K., Araujo, D., Haegelen, C., Collins, D.L.: Online database of clinical MR and ultrasound images of brain tumors. Medical Physics 39, 3253 (2012)
3. Collins, D.L., Zijdenbos, A., Kollokian, V., Sled, J., Kabani, N., Holmes, C., Evans, A.: Design and construction of a realistic digital brain phantom. IEEE Trans. Medical Imag. 17, 463–468 (1998)
4. http://scholar.google.ca/citations?view_op=view_citation&hl=en&user=ib5GlrQAAAAJ&citation_for_view=ib5GlrQAAAAJ:u-x6o8ySG0sC
5. Jensen, J.A.: Field: A program for simulating ultrasound systems. In: 10th Nordicbaltic Conference on Biomedical Imaging, vol. 4 (suppl.1), part 1, pp. 351–353. Citeseer (1996)
6. Jensen, J.A.: A model for the propagation and scattering of ultrasound in tissue. The Journal of the Acoustical Society of America 89, 182 (1991)
7. Afsham, N., Najafi, M., Abolmaesumi, P., Rohling, R.: A generalized correlation-based model for out-of-plane motion estimation in freehand ultrasound (2013)
8. Hedrick, W.R., Hykes, D.L., Starchman, D.E.: Ultrasound physics and instrumentation. Mosby St. Louis (1995)
9. Mercier, L., Fonov, V., Haegelen, C., Del Maestro, R.F., Petrecca, K., Collins, D.L.: Comparing two approaches to rigid registration of three-dimensional ultrasound and magnetic resonance images for neurosurgery. International Journal of Computer Assisted Radiology and Surgery 7, 125–136 (2012)
10. Coupé, P., Hellier, P., Morandi, X., Barillot, C.: 3D rigid registration of intraoperative ultrasound and preoperative mr brain images based on hyperechogenic structures. Journal of Biomedical Imaging 1 (2012)
11. Nabavi, A., Black, P., et al.: Serial intraoperative magnetic resonance imaging of brain shift. Neurosurgery 48, 787–798 (2001)
12. Wachinger, C., Klein, T., Navab, N.: The 2D analytic signal for envelope detection and feature extraction on ultrasound images. Medical Image Analysis 16, 1073–1084 (2012)
13. Dumpuri, P., Thompson, R.C., Dawant, B.M., Cao, A., Miga, M.I.: An atlas-based method to compensate for brain shift: Preliminary results. Medical Image Analysis 11, 128–145 (2007)
14. Rivaz, H., Boctor, E.M., Choti, M.A., Hager, G.D.: Real-time regularized ultrasound elastography. IEEE Transactions on Medical Imaging 30, 928–945 (2011)
15. Mohana Shankar, P., Dumane, V., Reid, J.M., Genis, V., Forsberg, F., Piccoli, C.W., Goldberg, B.B.: Classification of ultrasonic b-mode images of breast masses using nakagami distribution. IEEE Transactions on Ultrasonics, Ferroelectrics and Frequency Control 48, 569–580 (2001)
16. Seabra, J., Sanches, J.: Modeling log-compressed ultrasound images for radio frequency signal recovery. In: 30th Annual International Conference of the IEEE, Engineering in Medicine and Biology Society (EMBS 2008) (2008)

Visual Odometry in Stereo Endoscopy by Using PEaRL to Handle Partial Scene Deformation*

Miguel Lourenço[1], Danail Stoyanov[2], and João P. Barreto[1,3]

[1] Institute of Systems and Robotics, University of Coimbra, Coimbra, Portugal
{miguel,jpbar}@isr.uc.pt
[2] Centre for Medical Image Computing, University College of London, London, UK
danail.stoyanov@ucl.ac.uk
[3] Perceive 3D, Coimbra, Portugal

Abstract. Stereoscopic laparoscopy provides the surgeon with the depth perception at the surgical site to facilitate fine micro-manipulation of soft-tissues. The technology also enables computer-assisted laparoscopy where patient specific models can be overlaid onto laparoscopic video in real-time to provide image guidance. To maintain graphical overlay alignment of image-guides it is essential to recover the camera motion and scene geometry during the procedure. This can be performed using the image data itself, however, despite of the mature state of structure-from-motion techniques, their application in minimally invasive surgery remains a challenging problem due non-rigid scene deformation. In this paper, we propose a method for recovering the camera motion of stereo endoscopes through a multi-model fitting approach which segments rigid and non-rigid structures at the surgical site. The method jointly optimizes the segmentation of image and uses the rigid structure to robustly estimate the motion of the laparoscope. Synthetic and *in-vivo* experiments show that the proposed algorithm outperforms RANSAC-based stereo visual odometry in non-rigid laparoscopic surgery scenes.

1 Introduction

Stereo laparoscopes are becoming increasingly popular in Minimally Invasise Surgey (MIS). The main reason behind their wide adoption is the possibility of recovering the 3D structure of the surgical site to provide the surgeon with depth perception of the operating field. Despite of being a difficult problem due to the dynamics of the medical environment that combine occlusions from the surgical instruments with strong specularities, several authors have already

---

* Miguel Lourenço and João Barreto want to thank *QREN-Mais Centro* by funding through the project *Novas Tecnologias para apoio à Saúde e Qualidade de Vida, Projecto A- Cirurgia e Diagnóstico Assistido por Computador Usando Imagem* and the Portuguese Science Foundation by funding through grant SFRH/BD/63118/2009. Danail Stoyanov thanks The Royal Academy of Engineering Research Fellowship for supporting his work.

C.A. Linte et al. (Eds.): AE-CAI 2014, LNCS 8678, pp. 33–40, 2014.

proposed efficient solutions for real-time computation of depth maps in medical endoscopy [1–3]. The obtained 3D structure can be used to align multimodal information [4] within a global reference 3D coordinate system [5] and enhance robotic instrument control.

An early work on structure-from-motion (SfM) in laparoscopic surgery was developed by Burschka *et al.* [5] where a rigid environment was assumed due to the confines of the sinus in order to compute a 3D scene map for registration with pre-operative Computed Tomography (CT) patient models. For procedures targeting soft-tissue anatomies non-rigidity due to cardiac, respiratory or peristaltic motions can make such SfM impossible. Deformable SfM (DSfM) [3], motion compensated SLAM [6] and more recently Non-Rigid SfM [7] have been proposed for overcoming this problem but an inspection phase to build a rigid template of the scene and strong priors deformation are not always feasible. For example motion and anatomical deformation due to instrument interactions cannot be reliably modelled prior to surgery and significant practical challenges remain for robust SfM in MIS. It is also possible to incorporate position sensors for additional constraints but this involves difficult integration solutions [8]. Close work to ours was proposed by Roussos *et al.* [9] that propose a multi-body segmentation framework with a direct hill climbing approach that alternates the estimation of region segmentation, camera motion, and depth. This results in a computationally heavy batch algorithm that requires a quite large number of frames to become feasible. Our paper shows that by recovering depth with stereo laparoscopy the problem is considerably simplified, and the region segmentation and camera motion estimation can be performed online as new data arrives.

This paper presents a solution to effectively segment non-rigid or piecewise rigid structures from the surgical site by using multi-model fitting [10]. To solve for the camera relative pose, we use a temporal clustering scheme to better distinguish which scene part should be used to anchor the camera motion estimation. When compared with the state-of-the-art in previously proposed solutions, our method does not require the entire scene to be rigid at an early inspection phase [11], being robust to parts that undergo non-rigid deformation while avoiding priors on these deformations [6]. Quantitative validation is performed with synthetic data [1] to illustrate the numerical stability and performance of the proposed method when the camera motion is accurately known. Qualitative validation in a long *in-vivo* video sequence shows that the proposed method is more effective in recovering the camera motion that the RANSAC-based state-of-the-art in stereo visual odometry [12].

2   Methods

Our method can be split in three main steps: (i) computing dense correspondences between two consecutive images; (ii) generating motion hypothesis using clustering of the motion field with a multi-model fitting approach; (iii) temporal consistency based segmentation of rigid structures that enable the recovery of the camera motion. These steps are described in detail in the sections below.

2.1   Disparity Computation and Pixel-to-Pixel Association

The stereo endoscopic images are assumed to be rectified for disparity map computation and the device is calibrated to determine the intrinsic and extrinsic camera parameters. Given a point $\mathbf{x}_l = (x_l, y_l)^{\mathsf{T}}$ on the left image I_l, the goal is to compute the projection of the same point on the right image I_r that is given by $\mathbf{x}_r = (x_l + d, y_l)$. Ideally, the disparity map D is built by computing d for every image pixel. For the disparity map computation we use the method proposed by Geiger *et al.* [2] that builds a prior over the disparity space by forming a triangulation on a set of robustly matched support points, and subsequently propagates structure into neighbouring image points.

For associating the disparity maps between two consecutive time instants $\mathsf{D}_l \leftrightarrow \mathsf{D}'_l$ we use a standard optical flow method [13] in 2D image space $\mathsf{I}_l \leftrightarrow \mathsf{I}'_l$. For computational reasons we do not compute the flow for every image pixel with a valid disparity and instead we sample the image space by using an equally spaced grid. Our criteria for sampling the grid is defined as function of image resolution to obtain ≈ 4000 point associations between frames.

2.2   Motion Hypothesis Clustering and Refinement with PEaRL

After computing the putative matches $\mathbf{x}_l \leftrightarrow \mathbf{x}'_l$, the correspondence in 3D space $\mathbf{X} \leftrightarrow \mathbf{X}'$ are obtained by using the corresponding disparity values. For registration of the 3D point clouds we use the absolute orientation method [14]. Because different motions can be present at the surgical non-rigid site, we apply the energy-based PEaRL algorithm for labelling the data points with the corresponding motion [10, 15]. This procedure involves three steps: (i) generate an initial set of motion hypotheses, (ii) inlier classification by using an assigned a label (rigid motion) to the putative matches, and (iii) motion refinement using the discrete label assignment.

We start by generating camera motion hypothesis $\mathsf{T} = [\mathsf{R}\ \mathbf{t}]$ by sampling sets of 3 neighbouring points (minimal case for [14]) without repetition. Up to 500 motion hypothesis with support larger than 1% the number of pixels on the sample grid are used. Given the set of motion hypothesis $\mathcal{T}$, the goal is to expand the models and estimate their support. This is achieved by applying PEaRL [10] to minimize the energy function

$$E(\mathbf{T}) = \underbrace{\sum_{\mathbf{x}} \mathcal{D}(\mathbf{x}, \mathsf{T}_{\mathbf{x}})}_{\text{Data cost}} + \lambda \underbrace{\sum_{(\mathbf{x},\mathbf{y}) \in \mathcal{N}} w(\mathbf{x},\mathbf{y}) \delta(\mathsf{T}_{\mathbf{x}}, \mathsf{T}_{\mathbf{y}})}_{\text{Smoothness term}} + \underbrace{\beta |\mathcal{T}_T|}_{\text{Label cost}} , \qquad (1)$$

where $\mathbf{T} = \{\mathsf{T}_{\mathbf{x}} | \mathbf{x} \in \mathbf{P}\}$ is an assignment of rigid motion models to data points $\mathbf{x} = \{\mathbf{x}_l, \mathbf{x}'_l\}$. The data cost term $\mathcal{D}(\mathbf{x}, \mathsf{T}_{\mathbf{x}})$ is the reprojection error [16] that enables to measure the error in 2D, which is more robust than directly compute the data cost in the 3D point clouds [12]. The second terms is a smoothness term that encourages the assignment of the same label (rigid motion) to spatially close points. For each data point $\mathbf{x}$ only its 10 nearest neighbours $\mathbf{y}$ are

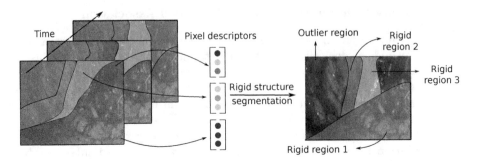

Fig. 1. Rigid segmentation algorithm. At each frame, one label is assigned to a point correspondence (same color represent the same label, and magenta represent the outlier label). While rigid structures tend to be classified with same labels in different views, piecewise rigid or non-rigid parts tend to fragment into different labels or be classified as outliers.

considered to compute the weight $w(\mathbf{x}, \mathbf{p})$. Since we want to enforce spatial consistency in the segmentation we consider that closer points are more likely to be described by the same rigid motion, with the weight being inversely proportional to their euclidean distance. This achieved with the Gaussian function $w(\mathbf{x}, \mathbf{y}) = \exp\left(-\|\mathbf{x} - \mathbf{y}\|_2 / \sigma^2\right)$. $\delta(.)$ represent the Potts model, being 1 when $\mathsf{T}_\mathbf{x} \neq \mathsf{T}_\mathbf{y}$, and 0 otherwise [10, 15]. The label cost penalizes the number of different labels being assigned to the data points to avoid excessive fragmentation. To the possible set of rigid motions $\mathcal{T}$ we add an empty label $\emptyset$, which as a constant data cost of 1.5 pixels for all data point and label cost equal to zero. Occlusions and non-rigid tool-tissue interactions will be intrinsically handled by the outlier. The outlier label also enables to handle erroneous flow estimation and disparity values, avoiding the need to perform the flow (section 2.1) on a temporal window.

After the first label expand, the motion parameters are refined by using the inliers of each label. This is accomplished by minimizing the reprojection error [16] with the Levenberg-Marquardt algorithm [10,16], with the empty labels being discarded. The new set of labels is then used in a new expansion step with the algorithm iterating between labelling and motion refinement until the optimization does not decrease the energy of Eq. 1 or a certain number of iterations is reached. The constants λ and β were set to $\lambda = 1$ and $\beta = 200$. These values were empirically obtained, and were used across all the experiments.

2.3   Segmenting Multi-view Consistently Labelled Parts

The minimization of the energy function of Eq. 1 guaranties that a label is assigned to each data point $\mathbf{x}$. Since between two consecutive frames the non-rigid or piecewise rigid structures can be subtle and easily confused with the rigid ones, we adopt a window-based system where several frames are used to effectively distinguish between rigid and non-rigid scene parts.

Given a temporal window (see Fig. 1), we build a label-based descriptor for each pixel by concatenating the labels assigned in the frame-to-frame PEaRL optimization. Pixel descriptors with the outlier label assigned in one or more frames are discarded from further processing. The temporal segmentation is carried by clustering pixels with the exact same descriptor. In case of existing more than one cluster, the one with largest spatial support is selected as dominant rigid region and it is used to anchor the relative camera motion. Intuitively, we explore the fact that rigid structures tend to be classified with same labels in different views, while the piecewise rigid or non-rigid parts tend to fragment into different labels or be classified as outliers by the PEaRL algorithm.

Finally, bundle adjustment [16] is used to refine both the camera motion and the scene structure by using only the dominant rigid part of the scene. This step is necessary because non-rigid regions can contribute on a frame-to-frame basis (locally rigid) to the optimization with PEaRL. Ideally, the temporal segmentation could be computed in automatic manner for adapting to the magnitude of the deformation present in the scene, but this is means deterministic running times would be difficult to guarantee. In practice, we found that the 4/5 frames are sufficient to deal with large deformations and more subtle deformations.

3   Experiments and Results

For validation of the proposed method we conduct experiments with synthetic and *in-vivo* data. The proposed method was fully implemented in MATLAB, with exception of PEaRL which is implemented in C++ code [10]. The single core implementation of the algorithm runs at 0.5 fps in 960×540 images on an Intel i7-3630QM CPU @ 2.40GHz processor. Our method is compared with the RANSAC-based approach of [12] which is among the state-of-the art in visual odometry. This method is implemented in C++ and it runs at 2.5 fps after tuning the method parameters to obtain the best possible camera motion estimations.

3.1   Experiments in Synthetic Data

Camera and scene motion ground truth is difficult to obtain for *in-vivo* MIS video and therefore, the proposed method is validated in a synthetic environment for which the camera motion is precisely known. While simulation sequences cannot render the full complexity of the surgical environment they allow to test the accuracy of the proposed method against different levels of white image noise to illustrate the numerical properties of the method. This sequence comprises 90 frames with the largest part of the scene ($> 60\%$) presenting strong deformation. Figure 2(b) shows the camera motion estimation in the noise free case. It can be seen that our trajectory closely follows the ground truth one, enabling accurate camera estimation in case of such large deformation, while Geiger's method [12] tends to follow the non-rigid deformation motion. Figures 2(c) and 2(d) shows the translation and rotation errors for increasing levels of image noise, showing that our method is numerically stable under moderate amounts of image noise.

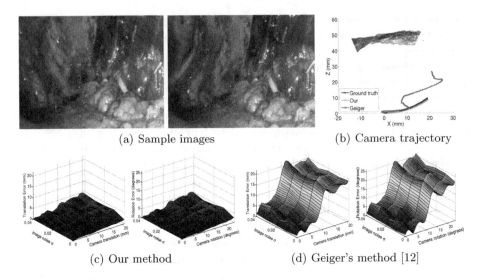

(a) Sample images   (b) Camera trajectory

(c) Our method   (d) Geiger's method [12]

Fig. 2. Simulation results under increasing level of image noise. (a) show the simulation images with large deformation between them. (b) show the camera trajectory estimation for the zero noise case. Green curve represent the ground truth, blue is ours, and red is obtained with Geiger's method. (c,d) show the performance of both methods under increasing amount of additive white noise. For each method, the left graphics show the translation error as a function of the camera translation motion and level of noise. The same is done for the rotation on the right. It can be seen that our method is numerically stable under moderate levels of image noise.

3.2 Experiments in *in-vivo* Data

The data used in this experiment was recorded with *da Vinci Si* surgical robot during a robotically assisted prostatectomy surgery. Our and Geiger's methods [12] were used to recover the camera motion and also the dense 3D scene reconstruction. This sequence of 500 frames is particularly challenging due to the presence of non-rigid motion, strong specularities, bleeding and physiological motion due to large vascular structures in the view. At the end the sequence the camera approximately returns to the starting point performing a loop-closure which can be used for qualitative assessment.

Figure 3 shows the results for camera motion estimation using our and Geiger's methods. Since our solution effectively segments the non-rigid parts of the scene, the camera motion is reliably recovered. Geiger's method employs a conventional frame-to-frame RANSAC-based approach that is less suitable for the challenges in MIS images with the trajectory clearly drifting in the presence of non-rigid motion. To provide a quantitative measure of the quality of the motion estimation, we compute the reprojection error of the reconstructed 3D points, where it can be seen that our method enables more accurate reconstruction and camera motion estimation. It can also be seen that our method is considerably more closer to perform the loop closing, with an error in position of $0.6\,mm$ and an

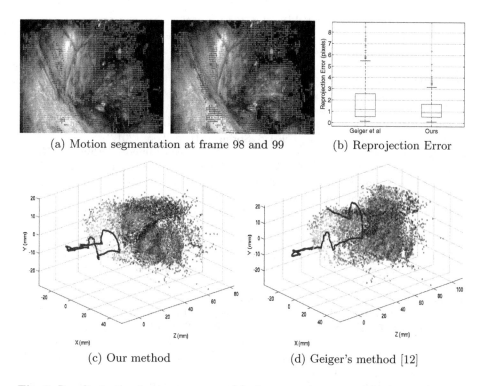

(a) Motion segmentation at frame 98 and 99   (b) Reprojection Error

(c) Our method   (d) Geiger's method [12]

Fig. 3. Results in the *in-vivo* sequence. (a) shows two instants with the overlay segmentation. Magenta represent the outlier label that increases with larger deformation. (b) shows the reprojection error obtained with each pixel in frame-by-frame basis. (c,d) show the results of our method and the method of [12] for the camera motion recovery. Our method is capable of performing reliable long-term camera motion estimation, while [12] tends to deteriorate the estimations due to the presence the non-rigid parts.

orientation error of 5.2 degrees, while the Geiger's method has an error in position of $28\,mm$ and an orientation error of 24.34 degrees.

4   Discussion and Conclusions

We have presented a method for rigid structure segmentation and camera motion estimation during stereoscopic MIS. The proposed method relies on PEaRL [10] for segmenting the scene rigid structures to anchor the camera motion estimation. Temporal consistency is enforced by clustering the segmented scene structures according to the labelling assigned in the PEaRL step. Quantitative and qualitative validation in simulation and *in-vivo* data show that our solution enables to keep accurate camera motion estimation in the presence of significant non-rigid deformation, outperforming a RANSAC-based state-of-the-art method in stereo visual odometry [12]. Future work includes the implementation of our solution for real-time stereo visual odometry using parallelization with GPGPU, and investigation of more suitable solutions for performing the correspondences directly in the 3D space by exploring stereoscopic flow [1].

References

1. Stoyanov, D.: Stereoscopic Scene Flow for Robotic Assisted Minimally Invasive Surgery. In: Ayache, N., Delingette, H., Golland, P., Mori, K. (eds.) MICCAI 2012, Part I. LNCS, vol. 7510, pp. 479–486. Springer, Heidelberg (2012)
2. Geiger, A., Roser, M., Urtasun, R.: Efficient Large-Scale Stereo Matching. In: Kimmel, R., Klette, R., Sugimoto, A. (eds.) ACCV 2010, Part I. LNCS, vol. 6492, pp. 25–38. Springer, Heidelberg (2011)
3. Maier-Hein, L., et al.: Optical techniques for 3d surface reconstruction in computer-assisted laparoscopic surgery. Medical Image Analysis 17, 974–996 (2013)
4. Roehl, S., et al.: Dense gpu-enhanced surface reconstruction from stereo endoscopic images for intraoperative registration. Medical Physics 39, 1632–1645 (2012)
5. Burschka, D., Li, M., Ishii, M., Taylor, R., Hager, G.: Scale-invariant registration of monocular endoscopic images to ct-scans for sinus surgery. Medical Image Analysis 9, 413–426 (2005)
6. Mountney, P., Yang, G.-Z.: Motion compensated slam for image guided surgery. In: Jiang, T., Navab, N., Pluim, J.P.W., Viergever, M.A. (eds.) MICCAI 2010, Part II. LNCS, vol. 6362, pp. 496–504. Springer, Heidelberg (2010)
7. Garg, R., Roussos, A., Agapito, L.: Dense variational reconstruction of non-rigid surfaces from monocular video. In: IEEE Conference on Computer Vision and Pattern Recognition, pp. 1272–1279 (2013)
8. Luo, X., Mori, K.: Robust Endoscope Motion Estimation Via an Animated Particle Filter for Electromagnetically Navigated Endoscopy. IEEE Transactions on Biomedical Engineering 61, 85–95 (2014)
9. Roussos, A., Russell, C., Garg, R., Agapito, L.: Dense multibody motion estimation and reconstruction from a handheld camera. In: IEEE International Mixed and Augmented Reality, pp. 31–40 (2012)
10. Isack, H., Boykov, Y.: Energy-based geometric multi-model fitting. International Journal of Computer Vision 97, 123–147 (2012)
11. Giannarou, S., Zhang, Z., Yang, G.Z.: Deformable structure from motion by fusing visual and inertial measurement data. In: IEEE/RSJ International Conference on Intelligent Robots and Systems, pp. 4816–4821 (2012)
12. Geiger, A., Ziegler, J., Stiller, C.: Stereoscan: Dense 3d reconstruction in real-time. In: IEEE Intelligent Vehicles Symposium, pp. 963–968 (2011)
13. Farnebäck, G.: Two-Frame Motion Estimation Based on Polynomial Expansion. In: Bigun, J., Gustavsson, T. (eds.) SCIA 2003. LNCS, vol. 2749, pp. 363–370. Springer, Heidelberg (2003)
14. Horn, B.K.P.: Closed-form solution of absolute orientation using unit quaternions. Journal of the Optical Society of America A 4, 629–642 (1987)
15. Boykov, Y., Veksler, O., Zabih, R.: Fast approximate energy minimization via graph cuts. IEEE Transactions on Pattern Analysis and Machine Intelligence 23, 1222–1239 (2001)
16. Triggs, B., McLauchlan, P.F., Hartley, R.I., Fitzgibbon, A.W.: Bundle adjustment – A modern synthesis. In: Triggs, B., Zisserman, A., Szeliski, R. (eds.) ICCV-WS 1999. LNCS, vol. 1883, pp. 298–375. Springer, Heidelberg (2000)

Instrument Tracking and Visualization
for Ultrasound Catheter Guided Procedures

Laura J. Brattain[1,2], Paul M. Loschak[1], Cory M. Tschabrunn[3], Elad Anter[3],
and Robert D. Howe[1]

[1] Harvard School of Engineering and Applied Sciences, Cambridge, MA USA
[2] MIT Lincoln Laboratory, Lexington, MA USA
[3] Harvard-Thorndike Electrophysiology Institute, Beth Israel Deaconess Medical
Center, Harvard Medical School, Boston, MA USA

Abstract. We present an instrument tracking and visualization system
for intra-cardiac ultrasound catheter guided procedures, enabled through
the robotic control of ultrasound catheters. Our system allows for rapid
acquisition of 2D ultrasound images and accurate reconstruction and
visualization of a 3D volume. The reconstructed volume addresses the
limited field of view, an inherent problem of ultrasound imaging, and
serves as a navigation map for procedure guidance. Our robotic system
can track a moving instrument by continuously adjusting the imaging
plane and visualizing the instrument tip. The overall instrument tracking
accuracy is $2.2mm$ RMS in position and $0.8°$ in angle.

Keywords: instrument tracking, intra-cardiac imaging, volume rendering, procedure guidance.

1   Introduction

Catheters enable many diagnostic and repair procedures to be accomplished with
minimal collateral damage to the patients healthy tissues. In complex catheter
procedures, workflow is often limited by visualization capabilities, which contributes to operator's inability to prevent and assess complications, as well as
facilitation of key procedural components. In electrophysiological (EP) cardiac
procedures, guidance is largely provided by fluoroscopy. However this imaging
modality is unable to image soft tissues. To compensate for this shortcoming,
a widely adopted approach is to generate a 3D electrophysiological model re-
sembling the shape of the cardiac chamber by using a magnetic position sensing
system that records the locations of the ablation catheter tip in space. The
point clouds of the catheter tip positions may then be registered to a CT or
MRI based pre-operative anatomical model and displayed to the clinician with
the real-time positions of the catheters superimposed [1, 2]. Although the acquisition of catheter based geometry is acquired in real-time, the registration
with pre-operative rendered anatomy is not, and thus may result in an anatomic
mismatch at the time of the procedure.

C.A. Linte et al. (Eds.): AE-CAI 2014, LNCS 8678, pp. 41–50, 2014.
© Springer International Publishing Switzerland 2014

Ultrasound (US) imaging catheters (intra-cardiac echocardiography, or ICE) have been routinely used in EP procedures for over a decade [3]. These catheters are inserted into the patients vasculature (e.g. femoral vein) and navigated to the heart, where they acquire B-mode images of cardiac structures. Compared to external probes, ICE can achieve higher quality views of targets in the near field with higher acoustic frequencies, reducing aberration and attenuation. The versatility of ICE imaging is particularly important during EP procedures, as it provides excellent visualization of all cardiac chambers when the probe is placed in the appropriate anatomic position. Recent studies suggest that ICE monitoring of lesion formation may increase the effectiveness of ablation procedure [3, 4].

Unfortunately, controlling ICE catheters requires the clinician to aim the imaging plane by manually turning control knobs and rotating and advancing the catheter handle. This makes it highly challenging to align the image plane with the target, thus moving between targets requires extensive time and skill to obtain an adequate view. During navigation of a working catheter based instrument, cardiologists presently use a combination of pre-operative images, fluoroscopic imaging, electroanatomic mapping, and minimal haptic feedback through the catheter handle. However, the actual instrument tip-to-tissue interaction can only be visualized in real-time with the use of US imaging, and these interactions could be effectively visualized with ICE. This presents a challenge for the operator because significant training and time are required to manually maneuver the ICE catheter. As a result, the use of ICE has largely been limited to a few critical tasks such as transseptal puncture.

We hypothesize that automatic tracking of the working instrument tool tip with direct visual feedback will better facilitate cardiac procedures such as ablation, including confirmation of adequate instrument tip-to-tissue contact. Real-time monitoring also enables rapid lesion assessment and may aid in the detection of impending complications. Automatic panoramic US imaging and enhanced displays also promise to decrease the need for fluoroscopy, reducing ionizing radiation exposure to patients and medical personnel. To our knowledge, no similar capability has been reported in the literature. Instrument tracking and real-time visual feedback using ICE are unique contributions of our system.

In this paper, we begin with an overview of the hardware of a robotic ICE steering system, which we previously developed. Next, we describe the imaging capabilities that we have developed for 3D mosaicing and instrument tracking, followed by experimental results. We conclude with a discussion of both the contributions and limitations of our current system.

2   System and Design

2.1   System Overview

We developed a robotic ICE control system to automate the pointing of ICE catheters. An ICE catheter, such as the one shown in Fig. 1, is a four degree-of-freedom (DOF) system that has two orthogonal bending directions and can translate along and rotate about its base axis. Our robotic manipulator has four motors, each controlling one of the four DOFs (Fig. 2). We derived and implemented a closed-form solution for forward and inverse catheter kinematics, which controls ICE tip position and imaging plane orientation [5]. An electromagnetic (EM) tracker system (trakSTAR, Ascension Technology, Shelburne, VT, USA) is used for closed loop control, performance validation, and safety functions.

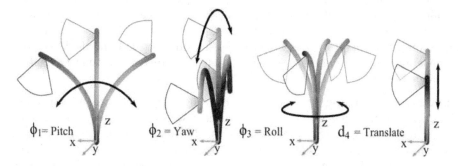

$\phi_1 =$ Pitch $\phi_2 =$ Yaw $\phi_3 =$ Roll $d_4 =$ Translate

Fig. 1. A schematic diagram showing the four degrees of freedom of an ICE catheter

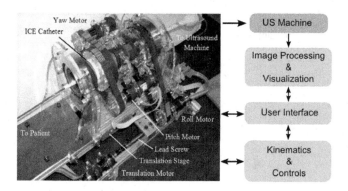

Fig. 2. System Overview. (*Left*) Robotic manipulator. (*Right*) System key modules and workflow.

2.2   System Capabilities

Safety is always a priority in a clinical environment, thus being able to perform imaging tasks while keeping the ICE catheter tip stationary is a useful capability. Based on this important assumption, we developed the following key capabilities:

Sweeping: Automated image plane sweeping adjusts the imager while keeping the ICE catheter tip at a fixed location to build a real-time 3D 'panorama' (Fig. 3(a)). This shows the tissue structure across a treatment area and beneath the surface. The sweeping capability is different from simply rotating the catheter handle or body around its rotational axis in that it actually uses a combination of three knob adjustments to rotate the imager about its distal tip. During manual manipulation, a clinician may wish to position the ICE catheter in a desired region of the heart and sweep the imaging plane to get a comprehensive view of the region. When the catheter tip is already in a bent configuration, it is extremely difficult to intuitively spin the catheter manually about its own axis while keeping the tip in place. In automated sweeping, the user may input the desired range of angles to sweep with a specified angular resolution. By combining position and roll control, the US transducer can be rotated to a desired angle while the tip is continuously position controlled to remain at a fixed point. Several sweeps can be done at a few different user specified locations to generate a large, patient specific anatomical map for real-time navigation guidance.

Instrument Tracking: In instrument tracking mode, the system can follow the tip of an instrument (e.g. ablation catheter). The robot aims the imaging plane at a moving target while keeping the ICE catheter tip at a fixed and safe location (Fig. 3(b)). This is achieved by computing the angle between the target and the ICE imaging plane and commanding a specific roll. The position controller makes small adjustments of the ICE catheter tip position during the roll to maintain the stationary position.

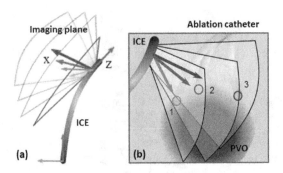

Fig. 3. Schematic illustration of system capabilities. (a) Sweeping. (b) Tracking ablation catheter tool tip.

2.3   3D Reconstruction of 2D ICE Images from Sweeping

The sweeping functionality enables the acquisition of closely spaced 2D images across a user specified region of interest (ROI). The 2D slices are non-parallel sections which need to be spatially registered to a common Cartesian coordinate frame using the tool tip positions acquired by the EM tracker and then interpolated and compounded into a gridded 3D volume. Fig. 4 shows the 3D panorama creation pipeline. There are several leading methods for 3D reconstruction of ultrasound images [6–10]. Our method is essentially the voxel-based interpolation.

In order to achieve real-time performance, we implemented the 3D stitching and visualization on a GPU based on our previous real-time mosaicing technique for 3D/4D ultrasound [11, 12].

The registered 2D slices typically are not well aligned with the gridded space, resulting in gaps in the reconstructed 3D volume. Fortunately, the 2D slices can be acquired at any spacing, so the gaps can be made small, at the expense of longer sweeping times. Furthermore, the actual catheter tip locations at two adjacent frames and the commanded tip trajectory are known. This allows us to generate an image through a 'virtual' tip position on the trajectory by projecting images from the two closest 2D frames to the virtual position. The new image is then interpolated onto the 3D volume. Coupe [13] reported a similar 3D freehand US reconstruction method using probe trajectory (PT), and concluded that since the virtual slice was generated by using the information from the closest two frames, this method outperformed traditional approaches such as Voxel Nearest Neighbor (VNN) [14] and Distance Weighted interpolation (DW) [15]. The main limitation of the PT method was the assumption of constant probe speed between two slices. This limitation does not exist in our system because the actual tip location and commanded trajectory are known.

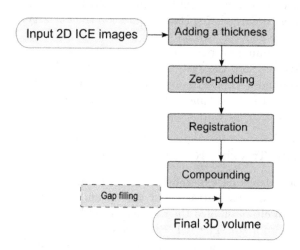

Fig. 4. 3D Panorama creation pipeline

3   Experimental Results

3.1   Sweeping

We conducted water tank experiments using gelatin-based phantoms that closely mimic the geometric and echogenic properties of animal tissue. The ICE catheter was connected to a Siemens Acuson X300 US imaging system and introduced through the side of the water tank where the imaging phantom was located.

The first experiment was to sweep across a specified ROI and build a 3D panorama. The imaging phantom was shaped to resemble the left atrium with four openings that simulate the pulmonary vein ostia (PVO), which are the critical areas for imaging during an atrial fibrillation ablation procedure. The atrium area (the opening in the phantom) was roughly $40m \times 40mm$. The ICE tip was directly in front of the phantom (Fig. 5(a)). The images were acquired at $90mm$ depth and $6.7MHz$ frequency. The system swept across the phantom in $1°$ increments over $40°$ while the ICE tip position remained stationary. Volume rendering was done as described in Sec. 2.3. Fig. 5(b)-(d) shows the reconstructed volume in three views. The PVOs are easily seen from Fig. 5(c).

To compute the reconstruction accuracy, features along the sweeping trajectory were measured and compared to their actual dimensions. Phantom atrium width and the length of two PVO vessels were manually determined in QLAB (Philips Healthcare, Andover, MA) in 20 images. Corresponding physical ground truth values were obtained by caliper measurements ($\pm 0.25mm$). Analysis shows that system accuracy is $0.96mm$ RMS (range $0.68 - 1.3mm$).

To register and interpolate one 2D ICE image into the 3D volume requires $30ms$. Volume reconstruction time depends on the sweep angle and resolution. For instance, the total reconstruction time on GPU for a dense sweep of 40 images takes approximately $1.5s$. Data acquisition time is largely determined by the robotic system and the cardiac rate. Each $1°$ step is done in roughly $2s$, roughly twice the minimum possible due to heart rate (assuming a heart rate of 60 BPM). At each step the system must pause to acquire images across the cardiac cycle to build a 4D panorama. The total panorama creation time is 1-2 minutes, much less than the time for model building with clinical EP systems such as Ensite NavX [1] or CartoSound [2].

3.2   Instrument Tracking Results

In the instrument tracking experiment, the instrument was a $3mm$ diameter catheter with an EM sensor attached at the tip and calibrated to the catheter tip position. It closely resembled the dimensions and echogenic properties of an ablation catheter tool tip. The ICE catheter tracked the tool tip as it moved around the simulated PVO in the atrium phantom. Fig. 6(a) shows the experiment setup and Fig. 6(b) plots the imaging plane x-axis as it followed the tool tip. The lines show a top-view of imaging planes and the circles represent tool tip positions. Colors indicate corresponding imaging planes and tool tip positions. Fig. 6(c) is an example 2D ICE image during instrument tracking.

We also conducted an instrument tracking accuracy analysis study. Fig. 7(a) is a plot of the histogram of ICE imaging plane to tool tip distance. It shows that during majority of the trials, the tool tip is within $1 - 2mm$ from the imaging plane, thus it appears in the image. Fig. 7(b) is the histogram of ICE imaging plane pointing angular error. The average angular error is $0.3°$, and the maximum error is below $0.5°$. When including the EM tracker angular error ($0.5°$ RMS in angle [16]), the overall system angular tracking accuracy is $0.8°$.

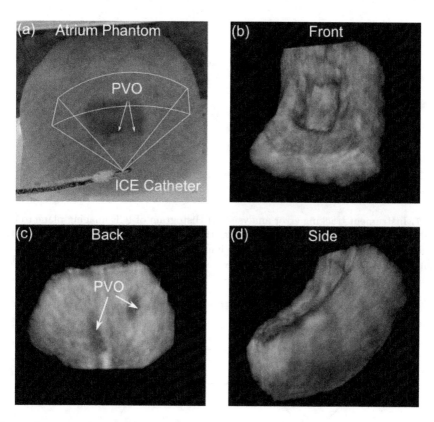

Fig. 5. Sweeping results. (a) Atrium phantom. (b)-(d) Mosaiced volume of the atrium phantom from three different views. The phantom PVO can be clearly seen from (c).

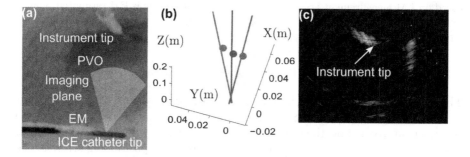

Fig. 6. Instrument tracking. (a) Instrument tip at simulated PVO. (b) Typical trajectory of imaging plane following the tool tip when looking top down from the imaging plane x-axis. The lines show imaging plane x-axis, the circles represent tool tip positions. Colors indicate corresponding imaging planes and tool tip positions. (c) Example 2D ICE image during instrument tracking.

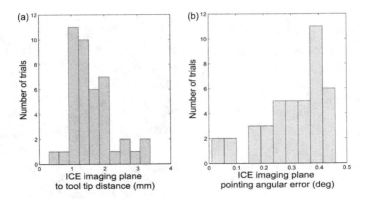

Fig. 7. Instrument tracking error analysis. (a) Histogram of ICE imaging plane to tool tip distance. During majority of the trials, the tool tip is within $1 - 2mm$ from the imaging plane, thus the tip appears in the image. (b) Histogram of ICE imaging plane pointing angular error. Average angular error is $0.3°$. The maximum error is below $0.5°$.

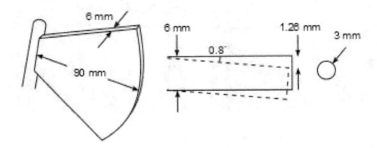

Fig. 8. Imaging plane thickness and tracking accuracy. (*Left*) Typical ICE imaging plane depth. (*Right*) cross section view of imaging plane for calculation of accuracy based on EM measurement accuracy of sweep angle: solid line is EM estimated boundary of image plane, dotted line is worst case scenario; circle is target ablation catheter cross section to show relative sizes.

3.3 ICE Imaging Plane Thickness vs. System Accuracy

The inaccuracy of the EM trackers in ICE and the working instrument may result in the misalignment of the US imaging plane with the instrument. In this case the image may not show the tool tip. To analyze accuracy limits, the thickness of the ICE imaging plane can be compared to the possible positioning errors of the tool tip. Fig. 8 illustrates a simplified case considering only misalignment error in the sweep angle, using a typical ICE image plane depth $90mm$ and thickness $6mm$ [17].

RMS accuracy specifications for the EM tracker are $1.4mm$ in position and $0.5°$ in angle [16] and our system tracking accuracy is $0.3°$. A simple geometric analysis of the worst-case accuracy scenario shows that an ablation catheter of diameter $3mm$ would be visible in the US image, although it may not be in the mid-plane. EM interference in clinical procedure rooms will likely decrease the accuracy of the EM trackers, although the close proximity of the imaging catheter to the ablation catheter will minimize the relative tracking errors.

4   Discussion and Conclusion

This is the first paper to demonstrate that robotic steering of an ICE catheter can produce high quality volumetric image and tracking is accurate enough to visualize moving instruments. The system manipulates floppy, deformable off-the-shelf ICE catheters, which are challenging to navigate manually. Our previous paper ([5]) detailed only the robot while this paper focuses on the imaging results, which have not been presented before.

Situational awareness plays a critical role in intra-operative procedure guidance. The current environment lacks real-time direct visual feedback of instrument-tissue interactions, which in part contributes to the low success rate of ablation procedures. The system presented in this paper addresses this issue with the following capabilities: (1) Build a real-time panorama of a ROI by spinning ICE at desired angles while keeping its tip at a fixed and safe location; (2) Instrument tracking and image-based tip location identification. Both tasks would be difficult to achieve manually. Our system can be easily extended to 4D (3D + time) based on our previous work on 4D US mosaicing and visualization with ECG gating [11, 12]. In addition to better spatial localization when compared to 2D views, the reconstructed 3D volume can also be used for surface and instrument segmentation, which would facilitate the integration with current clinical EM mapping systems or with an augmented virtual reality environment.

We believe our robotic system in combination with US image processing and visualization capabilities has the potential to further improve intra-operative procedure guidance.

Acknowledgments. MIT Lincoln Laboratory work is sponsored by the Department of the Air Force under Air Force contract #FA8721-05-C-0002. Opinions, interpretations, conclusions and recommendations are those of the authors and are not necessarily endorsed by the United States Government. Harvard University work is supported by the US National Institutes of Health under grant NIH R01 HL073647.

References

1. Ensite: Ensite navx cardiac mapping system. st. jude medical (July 2014), http://professional.sjm.com/products/ep/mapping-visualization/cardiac-mapping-system
2. CartoSound: Biosense webster (March 2014), http://www.biosensewebster.com/cartosound.php

3. Marrouche, N.F., Martin, D.O., Wazni, O., Gillinov, A.M., Klein, A., Bhargava, M., Saad, E., Bash, D., Yamada, H., Jaber, W.: Phased-array intracardiac echocardiography monitoring during pulmonary vein isolation in patients with atrial fibrillation impact on outcome and complications. Circulation 107(21), 2710–2716 (2003)

4. Wright, J., Pless, R.: Analysis of persistent motion patterns using the 3d structure tensor. In: Seventh IEEE Workshops on Application of Computer Vision, WACV/MOTIONS 2005, vol. 1, 2, pp. 14–19. IEEE (2005)

5. Loschak, P.M., Brattain, L.J., Howe, R.D.: Automated pointing of cardiac imaging catheters. In: Proc. IEEE Int. Conf. Robotics and Automation (2013), NIHMS485450

6. Gee, A.H., Treece, G.M., Prager, R.W., Cash, C.J., Berman, L.: Rapid registration for wide field of view freehand three-dimensional ultrasound. IEEE Transactions on Medical Imaging 22(11), 1344–1357 (2003)

7. Prager, R., Ijaz, U., Gee, A., Treece, G.: Three-dimensional ultrasound imaging. Proceedings of the Institution of Mechanical Engineers, Part H: Journal of Engineering in Medicine 224(2), 193–223 (2010)

8. Rohling, R., Gee, A., Berman, L.: A comparison of freehand three-dimensional ultrasound reconstruction techniques. Medical Image Analysis 3(4), 339–359 (1999)

9. Barry, C., Allott, C., John, N., Mellor, P., Arundel, P., Thomson, D., Waterton, J.: Three-dimensional freehand ultrasound: image reconstruction and volume analysis. Ultrasound in Medicine & Biology 23(8), 1209–1224 (1997)

10. Solberg, O.V., Lindseth, F., Torp, H., Blake, R.E., Hernes, T.A.N.: Freehand 3d ultrasound reconstruction algorithms, a review. Ultrasound in Medicine & Biology 33(7), 991–1009 (2007)

11. Brattain, L.J., Howe, R.D.: Real-time 4D ultrasound mosaicing and visualization. In: Fichtinger, G., Martel, A., Peters, T. (eds.) MICCAI 2011, Part I. LNCS, vol. 6891, pp. 105–112. Springer, Heidelberg (2011)

12. Brattain, L.J., Vasilyev, N.V., Howe, R.D.: Enabling 3D ultrasound procedure guidance through enhanced visualization. In: Abolmaesumi, P., Joskowicz, L., Navab, N., Jannin, P. (eds.) IPCAI 2012. LNCS, vol. 7330, pp. 115–124. Springer, Heidelberg (2012)

13. Coupe, P., Hellier, P., Morandi, X., Barillot, C.: Probe trajectory interpolation for 3d reconstruction of freehand ultrasound. Medical Image Analysis 11(6), 604–615 (2007)

14. Prager, R.W., Gee, A., Berman, L.: Stradx: real-time acquisition and visualization of freehand three-dimensional ultrasound. Medical Image Analysis 3(2), 129–140 (1999)

15. Trobaugh, J.W., Trobaugh, D.J., Richard, W.D.: Three-dimensional imaging with stereotactic ultrasonography. Computerized Medical Imaging and Graphics 18(5), 315–323 (1994)

16. trakSTAR: Ascension (March 2014), http://www.ascension-tech.com/medical/trakSTAR.php

17. Zhong, H., Kanade, T., Schwartzman, D.: Image Thickness Correction for Navigation with 3D Intra-cardiac Ultrasound Catheter. In: Metaxas, D., Axel, L., Fichtinger, G., Székely, G. (eds.) MICCAI 2008, Part II. LNCS, vol. 5242, pp. 485–492. Springer, Heidelberg (2008)

Towards Video Guidance for Ultrasound, Using a Prior High-Resolution 3D Surface Map of the External Anatomy

Jihang Wang[1], Vikas Shivaprabhu[1], John Galeotti[1,2], Samantha Horvath[2], Vijay Gorantla[3], and George Stetten[1,2]

[1] Department of Bioengineering, University of Pittsburgh
[2] Robotics Institute, Carnegie Mellon University
[3] Department of Reconstructive Surgery, University of Pittsburgh Medical Center

Abstract. We are developing techniques for guiding ultrasound probes and other clinical tools with respect to the exterior of the patient, using one or more video camera(s) mounted directly on the probe or tool. This paper reports on a new method of matching the real-time video image of the patient's exterior against a prior high-resolution surface map acquired with a multiple-camera imaging device used in reconstructive surgery. This surface map is rendered from multiple viewpoints in real-time to find the viewpoint that best matches the probe-mounted camera image, thus establishing the camera's pose relative to the anatomy. For ultrasound, this will permit the compilation of 3D ultrasound data as the probe is moved, as well as the comparison of a real-time ultrasound scan with previous scans from the same anatomical location, all without using external tracking devices. In a broader sense, tools that know where they are by looking at the patient's exterior could have an important beneficial impact on clinical medicine.

Keywords: ultrasound, tracking, anatomical coordinates, computer vision, guidance, ProbeSight.

1   Introduction

Ultrasound (US) is an extremely useful clinical imaging modality for monitoring a wide variety of anatomical and physiological characteristics. It has numerous advantages including low-cost, real-time operation, portability, and lack of ionizing radiation. Whereas other image modalities such as computed tomography (CT) or magnetic resonance imaging (MRI) provide innate 3D anatomical coordinates, US scans lack such contextual correlates due to changing probe location. The operator holding the US probe may not feel this limitation during the scan, because the patient's external anatomy is clearly visible to provide navigational context. However, when reviewing the US images later, difficulties may arise in accurately interpreting the anatomical location, for example, to reposition the probe at precisely the same location and orientation with respect to the patient as a previous scan, or even simply

C.A. Linte et al. (Eds.): AE-CAI 2014, LNCS 8678, pp. 51–59, 2014.

to understand the underlying anatomy. Besides the ambiguity introduced by the freely moving probe, variation in joint pose as well as compression of tissue by the probe create serious challenges to interpreting US images not experienced with CT or MRI.

These challenges for US stem from its lack of a stable coordinate system. When assembling 3D US data from multiple 2D scans, the typical approach is to track the US probe relative to an external optical or magnetic tracking system, with the patient kept immobile during the scan. The external coordinate system of the tracker must then be related to the patient's anatomy to establish a context for the US scans. Our present research aims to replace such external tracking systems with a self-contained guidance system based on one or more video cameras mounted on the US probe itself. The camera's view of the external anatomy can provide anatomical coordinates for the US probe as it scans the patient. We call this self-contained guidance system *ProbeSight*, since it provides the US probe with a visual capability analogous to that of the human operator, to see for itself where it is relative to the patient.

Although the present paper mainly concerns our progress in using video to determine probe pose relative to external anatomy, we begin in Section 2 by describing how we will use that pose information to reconstruct and interrogate a 3D US data set. Our present reconstruction of 3D US employs conventional optical tracking, which we will eventually replace with the integrated video-based navigation system described in Section 3. Since the first clinical application intended for our system is monitoring patients after hand transplants, the anatomical target for our initial tests is the human forearm.

2   Reconstructing 3D Ultrasound Data Using External Tracking

One use for ProbeSight is to provide anatomical coordinates for reconstructing a 3D US dataset and retrieving arbitrary slices from it. A number of other researchers have developed systems to determine the US probe location using either optical or magnetic tracking systems, e.g. [1]. We have implemented a similar system, in which the location and orientation of the probe is determined by an external fixed optical tracking system (MicronTracker Sx60, Claron Technology) with a marker mounted on the US probe (Fig. 1A). We use this tracking system to reconstruct a 3D US dataset. For each B-scan, individual 2D images are stamped with the time of acquisition and the location of images obtained from the tracking system. A 3D volume is then reconstructed by placing the 2D images within a 3D space based on the tracking information (Fig. 1B). When the 2D images are consolidated into a 3D space, a particular voxel in the 3D volume may either be intersected by pixels from more than one 2D image or may not be intersected by any scan. As suggested in [2], the former problem, known as *bin-filling*, can be solved by combining data in the overlapping pixels (compounding). The latter problem, known as *hole-filling*, can be solved by inferring values for the missing data, using information of the voxel's neighbors (interpolation). We employ bin-filling and hole-filling techniques described in [3] and [4]. In order to correctly localize the data captured, temporal and spatial calibrations are required. We employ the method described in [5] for temporal calibration, to find the latency between the image acquisition and the tracking system. Spatial calibration finds the transformation between pixels in the 2D image and the location of the tracked marker on the probe in 3D space. We use an established N-wire phantom developed specifically for this purpose [6]. Our algorithms for calibration, image acquisition, and volume reconstruction are based on the Public Software Library for Ultrasound (PLUS) toolkit [7]. Reconstructed image slices that correspond to the current location of the US probe may then be retrieved from previously stored US data. To illustrate this, we use an US phantom containing tubing to simulate vasculature (Blue Phantom, Inc.). The phantom is tracked with reference markers. Fig 1D shows an image slice retrieved from a reconstructed 3D US volume of the phantom corresponding to the live US image seen in Fig 1C. The quality of the reconstructed slice suffers from the problems outlined above.

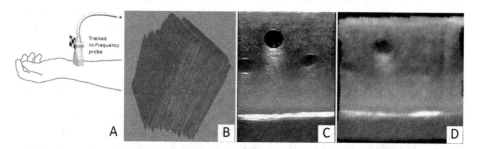

Fig. 1. (**A**) US probe tracked by markers mounted on it. (**B**) 3D model of individual 2D US images displayed in 3D space based on the recorded location and orientation of the US probe. (**C**) Live US image. (**D**) US image slice extracted from a previously reconstructed US volume corresponding to the live US image.

We have several reasons to want to replace external tracking systems in our application. Although they work well in a controlled environment, optical tracking demands continuous line of sight and magnetic tracking is unpredictable near ferromagnetic materials. Neither technology is generally as accurate as the vendors claim. Furthermore, an external tracking system restricts the portability of the US scanner, one of its great advantages in the hospital. Finally, the location of the patient and the particular anatomical target being scanned must be independently determined. ProbeSight addresses all of these problems.

3   Probe-Mounted Video Cameras to Replace the External Tracker

Attaching a video camera directly to the US probe theoretically permits determining the probe's pose relative to the patient's anatomy without any external tracking equipment. In [8] this approach was used to permit graphical overlays in the video image to show possible entry points for needle biopsy in the plane of the US scan. In [9] stereo cameras were mounted on the US probe to determine needle location relative to the probe. The US probe location relative to the patient's anatomy or US phantom has been determined by putting passive optical markers on the skin or phantom surface [10][11][12]. Such artificial surface markers can be problematic during clinical procedures, especially if they are to remain from one scan to the next. They may also influence the passage of US into patient and easily be smeared or distorted by the US gel. In our prior work we printed a checkerboard pattern on tracing paper and laid it upon a flat US phantom saturated with gel. The saturated tracing paper does not significantly interfere with the passage of US into the phantom, while remaining visible to stereo cameras mounted on the ultrasound probe, which determine the 3D location of the surface using stereo disparity [13].

We now propose to eliminate the optical trackers entirely and track natural skin features directly. The difficulties in applying computer vision algorithms to the unadulterated skin are significant. Hairless skin may contain only sparse features, hindering standard computer vision algorithms, such as stereo matching for determining depth, especially those algorithms operating without prior knowledge. We address this by providing detailed prior information in the form of a surface map, which we can match against images from the camera mounted on the ultrasound probe, close to the skin, where it can capture details such as pores and creases.

3.1   Using a High-Resolution Multi-camera Surface Map as Prior Information

We can greatly facilitate the determination of the probe-mounted camera's pose relative to the anatomy by supplying, beforehand, a detailed map of the entire anatomical terrain. Reconstructive surgeons already have devices with this ability. For example, the VECTRA M3 Imaging System (Canfield Imaging Systems) uses an array of three pairs of high-resolution cameras to acquire pre-operative images of anatomical structures for surgical planning. Over the course of several minutes, the system computes a detailed 3D surface map of the anatomy, including color texture with sufficient resolution to see pores and creases. Armed with such a prior scan, our probe-mounted camera can simply search for the matching portion of anatomy, much as a traveler might navigate with Google's Street View to stand in front of the correct house. We can render projections of the pre-acquired 3D surface map from any viewpoint to find a particular camera's actual viewpoint, and thus know the camera's pose relative to the external anatomy. Examples of projections of the surface map acquired from a subject's arm, rendered from three different viewpoints, are seen in Figure 2. Rather than match individual features, or small patches, as typical in stereo disparity routines, we will compare two entire images, a more robust proposition for computing camera pose.

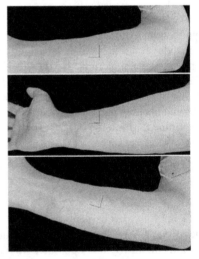

Fig. 2. Rendering a surface map from different viewpoints

3.2   Rendering the Surface Map as seen by a Real Camera

Rendering a 3D surface map to yield the particular 2D projection that would be seen by the probe-mounted camera requires more effort than typical of graphical rendering for entertainment or visualization purposes. The actual optics of the particular camera must be accurately modeled, including focal length, distortion, and location of entrance pupil. In addition, the simulated lighting applied during the rendering process should match the lighting during the acquisition of the surface map. We discuss each of these issues next.

   The 3D surface map data from the VECTRA imaging system consists of a tessellated point cloud, with every vertex assigned a color from the high-resolution camera array. We render this with OpenGL using a diffuse lighting model similar to the VECTRA scan's uniform lighting condition in the room where the VECTRA scanned the patient. Beyond the simple pinhole camera model used by OpenGL, however, we must model the optical parameters of our particular video camera.

   Distortions are inherent in any real lens design, and we model them as separate polynomial expansions in the radial and tangential directions. Radial distortion arises because the lens behaves differently at the center of the image than at the periphery, resulting in "barrel" or "pincushion" distortion. We characterize this by a Taylor series expansion around r, the distance from the image center. For typical optical lenses, we generally require only the first 2 terms, which are conventionally termed k_1 and k_2. For highly distorted optics such as fish-eye lenses it may be necessary to use a third radial distortion term k_3 [14]. Location (x, y) on the image sensor will thus be corrected according to the following equations:

$$x_{corrected} = x(1 + k_1r^2 + k_2r^4 + k_3r^6) \qquad y_{corrected} = y(1 + k_1r^2 + k_2r^4 + k_3r^6) \quad (1)$$

Tangential geometric distortion arises from imprecision during the manufacture of the camera resulting in the lens not being exactly parallel to the imaging plane. This can be minimally characterized by two additional parameters, p_1 and p_2, as follows [15]:

$$x_{corrected} = x + [2p_1y + p_2(r^2 + 2x^2)] \quad y_{corrected} = y + [2p_2x + p_1(r^2 + 2y^2)] \qquad (2)$$

All of these parameters can be estimated for a given camera, by applying existing routines in the Open-source Computer Vision (OpenCV) library to images taken by the camera of a standardized printed checkerboard pattern.

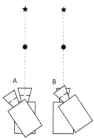

Fig. 3. Rotation to find entrance pupil

In addition to calibrating the camera, we also perform a physical alignment along the camera's depth axis in order to align the physical axis of rotation with the camera's entrance pupil. The entrance pupil is the point about which the camera can be rotated without changing the relative pixel alignment between the objects at different distances. It is essential to know the entrance pupil's physical location to determine the camera's location, and thus the US probe's location. Our strategy to find the entrance pupil is to point the camera toward two objects that are positioned to perfectly overlap when the camera is facing directly toward them. The camera is then rotated. If the entrance pupil is not the same as the rotation point, the two objects will no longer overlap when the camera is rotated (Fig. 3A). We then move the camera on a slider until we find the location about which, when the camera is rotated, the two objects always overlap (Fig. 3B).

With the above parameters determined and the focal length provided by the camera-lens manufacturer, it is possible to render the 3D surface map simulating the image that would be seen by the camera from any possible point of view.

3.3   2D Matching

Once the surface map has been rendered from a given viewpoint, it must be compared with the real-time image from the probe-mounted camera. A number of appropriate metrics are available, including normalized correlation. This method, however, does not perform well when pixels in the foreground (surface anatomy) are combined with significant regions of background that do not match. Segmenting foreground objects from the background by thresholding depth in the surface map can improve the matching result. However, we have found that mutual information [16][17], based on the joint distribution between the two images, is more reliable for our purposes, since it can accommodate differences in background without prior segmentation. In particular, we use *normalized mutual information* as described in [18].

3.4   Finding the Best Match

Given a metric for matching the rendering of the surface map to the real-time camera image, we can theoretically find the best match among all the possible camera viewpoints. However, the search space is very large, encompassing 6 degrees of freedom (DOFs): 3 translations and 3 rotations, and performing this search in real time presents challenges beyond the present paper. For now, we only demonstrate the accuracy of our projection method and the specificity of our matching process.

4   Validation

To validate our projection and matching methods, we used a textured phantom, in the form of a model dinosaur, roughly the same size as a human arm, viewed at a distance of approximately 20 cm. Note that in the eventual clinical system we expect the camera mounted on the US probe to be closer to the patient's skin, where finer details will be visible. We established ground truth for the location of the camera with respect to the dinosaur phantom using the same Micron optical tracking system described in Section 2. Markers for the tracking system were attached to a video camera (Prosilica GT1290C, Allied Vision Technologies) and the transformation between these markers and the cameras viewpoint determined, including entrance pupil. No US probe was included at this point. Five fiducials (small white dots) were painted on the surface of the phantom and a preassembled marker probe (Micron 950-MT-tool-B20) used to locate them in 3D space with the Micron tracker. These fiducials were also identified in the pre-acquired surface map using software for manually interrogating 3D data (MeshLab). Given this ground truth, we were able to predict the correct projection of the surface map to render, to match the actual image from the camera. An example of such a match is shown in Figure 4.

We tested the accuracy of our ground truth and the suitability of our metric by deviating along each of the six DOFs from the ground truth viewpoint, projecting the surface map from each new viewpoint and applying the metric between it and the actual camera

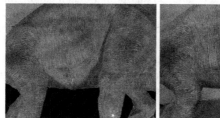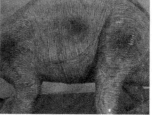

Fig. 4. Dinosaur model: Pre-acquired surface map (left), rendered from the correct viewpoint, matching the actual camera image (right). White dot fiducial on back leg.

image. With an image size of 640 × 480 pixels, a displacement of 1 pixel corresponds to approximately 1 mm at a range of 20 cm to the phantom. Results are shown in Figure 5, with ground truth marked by the vertical line in the middle of the range for each DOF. Along each DOF, the normalized mutual information metric shows a clear maximum at the ground truth viewpoint established by the tracking apparatus, and diminishes nearly monotonically as one moves away from the optimal pose.

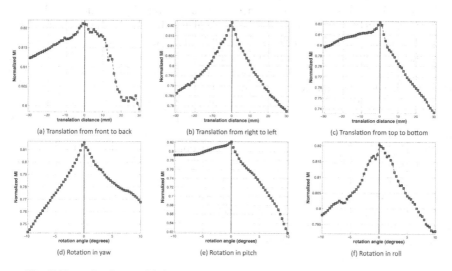

Fig. 5. Normalized mutual information for deviations from ground truth in each DOF

5   Discussion

We have established that we can project a previously acquired surface map of a phantom to match the view through an actual camera, and that mutual information is an effective metric to determine which viewpoint best matches the camera image.

Our next step is to develop efficient optimization routines to search the 6 DOFs for the maximum metric value, so that (1) an initial match can be obtained without the use of fiducial markers, and (2) an optimal match can be maintained in real time with further motion of the camera. The challenge of efficiently searching the 6-dimensional space needs to be addressed, and motion simultaneously in multiple DOFs must be accommodated.

Once a fully self-contained camera navigation system is functional and validated on the phantom, we will move to human subjects, beginning with the arm, to determine the robustness of the system on skin. We expect the finer detail of an arm compared to the dinosaur phantom to be visible given the closer range of the camera mounted on an actual ultrasound probe. We will still use the optical tracking apparatus for validation purposes, although it will eventually not be needed in the clinical system. With the camera attached to an actual US probe, we will adapt the US processing described in Section 2 so that ProbeSight provides the pose relative to the anatomy.

A major source of error in the matching process is the difference in lighting between the projected surface map and actual camera image. These differences may be reduced by controlling the lighting conditions during the pre-operative scan as well as during the actual scan, and by simulating correct lighting conditions when rendering the surface map using OpenGL lighting models. Attaching a lighting source to the probe itself is a possibility, especially given that ultrasound scans are often performed in a darkened or shadowy environment.

Tissue deformation is a major concern for any clinically practical ProbeSight system. We hope to be able to determine deformation by how far the location of the probe tip is computed to be beneath surface of the pre-acquired model. We also plan to include deformable registration, to accommodate deformation in the 2D matching process. Finally, we expect to incorporate analysis of the ultrasound data itself to detect in-slice deformation, such as demonstrated in [19].

The major contribution described in this paper is the use of a previously acquired high-resolution 3D surface map, against which a real-time camera image can be matched to provide anatomical coordinates for an ultrasound probe or surgical tool to which the camera is mounted. Such a technology could enable safe, economical, non-invasive, reliable and reproducible 3D visualization of intricate anatomy, providing spatial orientation and precise localization of structures such as vessels, nerves, tendons, muscle and bone without the limitations and risks of CT angiography, intravascular ultrasound or MRI. The applications of such a technology could span screening, diagnostic, therapeutic, interventional and management strategies, in a wide array of medical and surgical indications.

Acknowledgments. This work was funded by NIH R01 grant 1R01EY021641, National Library of Medicine contract HHSN276201000058OP, and Peer Reviewed Medical Research Program (PR130773, HRPO Log No. A-18237) award from the U.S. Department of Defense.

References

1. Flaccavento, G., Lawrence, P., Rohling, R.: Patient and probe tracking during freehand ultrasound. In: Barillot, C., Haynor, D.R., Hellier, P. (eds.) MICCAI 2004. LNCS, vol. 3217, pp. 585–593. Springer, Heidelberg (2004)

2. Rohling, R., Gee, A., Berman, L.: A comparison of freehand three-dimensional ultrasound reconstruction techniques. Medical Image Analysis 3(4) (1999)

3. Dewi, D., Wilkinson, M., Mengko, T., Purnama, I., van Ooijen, P., Veldhuizen, A., et al.: 3D Ultrasound Reconstruction of Spinal Images using an Improved Olympic Hole-Filling Method. In: ICICI-BME (2009)

4. Gobbi, D.G., Peters, T.M.: Interactive intra-operative 3D ultrasound reconstruction and visualization. In: Dohi, T., Kikinis, R. (eds.) MICCAI 2002, Part II. LNCS, vol. 2489, p. 156. Springer, Heidelberg (2002)

5. Rousseau, F., Hellier, P., Barillot, C.: A novel temporal calibration method for 3-D ultrasound. IEEE Transactions on Medical Imaging 25, 1108–1112 (2006)

6. Chen, T., Thurston, A., Ellis, R., Abolmaesumi, P.: A real-time freehand ultrasound calibration system with automatic accuracy feedback and control. Ultrasound in Medicine & Biology 35, 79–93 (2009)

7. Lasso, A., Heffter, T., Pinter, C., Ungi, T., Fichtinger, G.: Implementation of the PLUS open-source toolkit for translational research of ultrasound-guided intervention systems. The MIDAS Journal - Systems and Architectures for Computer Assisted Interventions Workshop, MICCAI, 1–12 (2012)

8. Khamene, A., Sauer, F.: Video-assistance for ultrasound guided needle biopsy. US Patent 6,612,991 (2002)

9. Chan, C., Lam, F., Rohling, R.: A needle tracking device for ultrasound guided percutaneous procedures. Ultrasound in Medicine & Biology 31(11) (2005)

10. Rafii-Tari, H., Abolmaesumi, P., Rohling, R.: Panorama ultrasound for guiding epidural anesthesia: A feasibility study. In: Taylor, R.H., Yang, G.-Z. (eds.) IPCAI 2011. LNCS, vol. 6689, pp. 179–189. Springer, Heidelberg (2011)

11. Sun, S., Anthony, B.: Freehand 3D ultrasound volume imaging using a miniature-mobile 6-DOF camera tracking system. In: 9th IEEE International Symposium (2012)

12. Sun, S., Gilbertson, M., Anthony, B.: 6-DOF probe tracking via skin mapping for freehand 3D ultrasound. In: 10thIEEE International Symposium (2013)

13. Wang, J., Horvath, S., Stetten, G., Siegel, M., Galeotti, J.: Real-Time Registration of Video with Ultrasound using Stereo Disparity. In: SPIE Medical Imaging, San Diego, CA (2012)

14. Fryer, J., Brown, D.: Lens distortion for close-range photogrammetry. Photogrammetric Engineering and Remote Sensing 52(1), 51–58 (1986)

15. Brown, D.: Decentering Distortion of Lenses. Photometric Engineering 32(3), 444–462 (1966)

16. Viola, P., Wells III, W.M.: Alignment by maximization of mutual information. International Journal of Computer Vision 24(2), 137–154 (1997)

17. Li, W.: Mutual information functions versus correlation functions. Journal of Statistical Physics 60(5-6), 823–837 (1990)

18. Studholme, C., Hill, D., Hawkes, D.: An overlap invariant entropy measure of 3D medical image anlignment. Pattern Recognition (32), 71–86 (1999)

19. Krupa, A., Fichtinger, G., Hager, G.D.: Real-time tissue tracking with B-mode ultrasound using speckle and visual servoing. In: Ayache, N., Ourselin, S., Maeder, A. (eds.) MICCAI 2007, Part II. LNCS, vol. 4792, pp. 1–8. Springer, Heidelberg (2007)

Fusion of Inertial Sensing to Compensate for Partial Occlusions in Optical Tracking Systems

Changyu He[1,2], H. Tutkun Şen[1], Sungmin Kim[1], Praneeth Sadda[1], and Peter Kazanzides[1]

[1] Johns Hopkins University, Baltimore MD 21218, USA
[2] Beijing Institute of Technology, Beijing 100081, China
hechangyu425@gmail.com, pkaz@jhu.edu

Abstract. Optical tracking is widely used for surgical Augmented Reality systems because it provides relatively high accuracy over a large workspace. But, it requires line-of-sight between the camera and the markers, which can be difficult to maintain. In contrast, inertial sensing does not require line-of-sight but is subject to drift, which causes large cumulative errors, especially for the measurement of position. This paper proposes a sensor fusion approach to handle cases where incomplete optical tracking information, such as just the 3D position of a single marker, is obtained. In this approach, when the optical tracker provides full 6D pose information, it is used to estimate the bias of the inertial sensors. Then, as long as the optical system can track the position of at least one marker, that 3D position can be combined with the orientation estimated from the inertial measurements to recover the full 6D pose information. Experiments are performed with a head-mounted display (HMD) that integrates an optical tracker and inertial measurement unit (IMU). The results show that with the sensor fusion approach we can still estimate the 6D pose of the head with respect to the reference frame, under partial occlusion conditions. The results generalize to a conventional navigation setup, where the inertial sensor would be co-located with the optical markers instead of with the camera.

1 Introduction

We are investigating the use of a head-mounted display (HMD) for presenting navigation information during surgical procedures[1][8]. We implemented our prototype system by mounting an optical see-through HMD (Juxtopia LLC, Baltimore, MD) and a small, commercially-available optical tracking system (Micron Hx40, Claron Technology, Toronto, Canada) on a helmet, as shown in Fig. 1. Ultimately, we envision integrating cameras directly on the HMD to avoid this cumbersome setup. Our goal is not to display high-resolution preoperative images on the HMD, but rather to show simple graphics derived from the navigation information. For example, the navigation information can include models of the patient anatomy that are obtained from preoperative images, such

C.A. Linte et al. (Eds.): AE-CAI 2014, LNCS 8678, pp. 60–69, 2014.
© Springer International Publishing Switzerland 2014

as biopsy target points and tumor outlines. Figure 2 illustrates two possible augmentation strategies: (a) overlaying the preoperative model directly on the patient's anatomy, and (b) displaying a "picture-in-picture" (PiP) virtual view of a model of the surgical instrument with respect to the preoperative model. The first strategy has the advantage that it is not necessary to track the instruments because their positions relative to the target are shown in the augmented view. But, this strategy also introduces technical challenges, especially when using an optical see-through HMD. In particular, it requires accurate calibration of the HMD to the surgeon's eyes (which must be maintained during the procedure, even if the HMD slips) and is subject to "swimming" effects due to the unavoidable delay in rendering overlays. We therefore adopted the second approach, which adds the requirement to track the surgical instrument. In either case, it is necessary to track the surgeon's head so that the the graphics are displayed from an intuitive perspective. This extra tracking requirement would exacerbate the existing concerns with maintaining line-of-sight between the tracking system camera and the markers on the patient, surgical instrument, and surgeon's head. We therefore chose an "inside out" tracking approach, where the camera is mounted on the HMD, as widely done in the augmented reality community [2], [13], [9], [4], [3], [10].

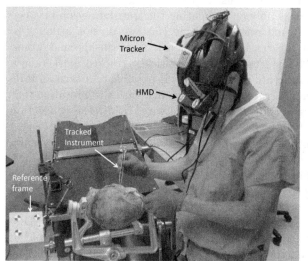

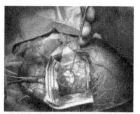

(a) Overlay on anatomy

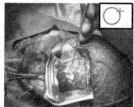

(b) PiP virtual view

Fig. 1. Cadaver experiment with head-mounted tracking system and display

Fig. 2. Conceptual illustrations of augmented views

We performed phantom experiments [8] and cadaver experiments (unpublished) in procedures emulating resection of convexity (brain surface) tumors. The HMD displayed the pose of the tracked surgical instrument with respect to 2D views of simulated tumor margins (in a real procedure, these would be segmented from preoperative CT or MRI images). As anticipated, mounting the camera on the surgeon's head avoided many line-of-sight issues because the surgeon typically did not block his own view of the patient. But, we discovered that it was difficult to keep the reference frame in the camera field of view because the head-mounted camera is much closer to the scene than an external camera mounted on a tripod or to the ceiling (see Fig. 1). One possible solution is to make a smaller reference frame, but that would reduce the accuracy of the orientation measurement. We therefore pursued a hybrid tracking approach, where we combined optical tracking and inertial sensing. Optical tracking provides drift-free measurement of position and orientation, but subject to a line-of-sight constraint and with slower update rates and higher latency. In contrast, inertial sensing (which includes accelerometers, gyroscopes, and magnetometers) provides low latency, high frequency measurements, but these sensors either provide derivatives of position/orientation and are subject to drift, or provide absolute orientation but are subject to disturbances (e.g., magnetometer). A sensor fusion approach enables us to take advantage of the strengths of each tracking technology [11].

We implement a Kalman Filter to estimate the orientation, but drive the system dynamics by the gyroscope and use the accelerometer and magnetometer to provide measurement updates. The camera always provides the position and, if the full marker frame is visible, the camera orientation is used to estimate the bias of the inertial sensors. Because we use a HMD, we place the IMU near the camera on the helmet and focus only on estimating the transformation between the surgeon's head (camera) and reference frame (i.e., we do not attempt to handle partial occlusion of the tracked instrument). But, the method would apply equally well if the IMU is attached to the optically-tracked markers in a more conventional navigation setup. In this case, it is possible to attach an IMU to each tracked device (reference frame and instrument), with the limitation that these devices cannot be passive and would require a wired or wireless connection to the measurement computer.

Fusion of inertial and optical sensing has been well studied in the literature, as in most of the augmented reality references cited above, but the goals have primarily been to: (1) provide more timely pose estimates than available with just optical tracking, (2) improve the accuracy of the data (especially the orientation), or (3) allow the system to continue to provide pose estimates if optical tracking is occluded for up to a few seconds. Our focus is to handle the situation where we have a partial occlusion of the optically-tracked markers; for example, if up to two of the markers on the Reference Frame in Fig. 1 are blocked. The partial occlusion case was previously addressed, with a different approach, by Tobergte[11], who used individual marker positions to correct the position and orientation estimated by an Extended Kalman Filter (EKF), with the system dynamics driven by the accelerometer and gyroscope feedback. Other researchers have handled partial occlusions by fusing optical and electromagnetic tracking systems [12]. The details of our approach are provided in the following sections.

2   Sensor Fusion Approach

The hybrid tracking unit contains one stereo camera (MicronTracker Hx40) and one IMU that is rigidly attached to the camera. The MicronTracker tracks special patterns at approximately 20 fps; the images are transferred to the host computer via a FireWire port. The IMU is a custom design with tri-axial accelerometer, gyroscope and magnetometer feedback. The 9 data values are provided to the host computer via a USB port; for the experiments in this paper, we used a data rate of 160 Hz. The two tracking units are registered by a calibration procedure [5]. The reference frame consists of three markers attached to a plastic board, as shown in Fig. 1. The reference frame is assumed to remain stationary during the procedure (more precisely, all other measurements are made relative to this frame so, without loss of generality, it can be assumed to be stationary). The test setup also includes a surgical instrument ("tool") that contains three tracked markers, though in a smaller physical arrangement (see Fig. 1). Our method does not handle occlusion or partial occlusion of the tool – if the marker frame is not visible, the tool model is not displayed in the augmented reality view. Note that tracking of the surgical instrument would not be required if the preoperative model were overlayed in-situ (on the anatomy), as in Fig. 2(a), which we believe would be more feasible with a video see-through HMD.

2.1   IMU Bias Estimation

The IMU provides three different types of three-axis measurements: (1) the gyroscope measures the angular rate of rotation, (2) the accelerometer measures the linear acceleration and the acceleration due to gravity, and (3) the magnetometer measures the earth's magnetic field (i.e., magnetic North).

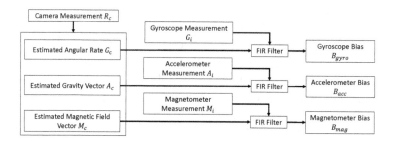

Fig. 3. Diagram of the bias calibration FIR filter

An optical tracking system can accurately track the position and orientation of objects within its field of view (FOV). We consider the optical tracker to be the ground truth and make the reasonable assumption that it does not contain a bias. Thus, we can use the output of the optical tracking unit to estimate the bias of the IMU sensors. Specifically, we used the cosine algorithm to calculate the true values A_{cn} and M_{cn} from the Euler angles obtained from the camera data. The bias can be estimated by subtracting these true values from the sensor feedback, and then using a Finite Impulse Response (FIR) filter to attenuate the noise, as shown in Fig. 3. This is given by the following equation, where the subscripts i and c indicate measurements from the IMU and camera, respectively, and a_n are the coefficients of the FIR filter ($\sum_n a_n = 1$):

$$
\begin{bmatrix} B_g \\ B_a \\ B_m \end{bmatrix} \approx \sum_n a_n \begin{bmatrix} G_{in} - G_{cn} \\ A_{in} - A_{cn} \\ M_{in} - M_{cn} \end{bmatrix}
\tag{1}
$$

The FDAtool was used to design the low pass FIR filter. Sampling frequency was 500, cutoff frequency was set as 20Hz and the order of the FIR filter was 20. This approach makes the following simplifying assumptions: (1) there is negligible acceleration, and (2) the latency between the IMU and optical tracker measurements is negligible. Both of these assumptions are satisfied under quasi-static conditions, where the surgeon's head is not moving very much.

2.2   Orientation Estimation

We use a Kalman Filter (KF) to estimate orientation from IMU sensor feedback, as illustrated in Fig. 4. Our state consists of a unit quaternion that represents the orientation. We use a discrete-time state equation that describes the evolution of the system state X_k, starting from the system state at the previous step X_{k-1} with the evolution law described by the matrix A and responding to system inputs u_k with the evolution law B.

$$
\hat{X}_k^- = A_k \hat{X}_{k-1} + Bu_k
\tag{2}
$$

The discrete-time matrix A_k has the following form, where $Gx(k)$, $Gy(k)$, and $Gz(k)$ are the angular velocities measured by the gyroscope, after removing the bias terms:

$$
A_k = \begin{bmatrix} 1 & -Gy(k)*t & -Gx(k)*t & -Gz(k)*t \\ Gy(k)*t & 1 & Gz(k)*t & -Gx(k)*t \\ Gz(k)*t & -Gy(k)*t & 1 & -Gx(k)*t \\ Gx(k)*t & Gy(k)*t & -Gz(k)*t & 1 \end{bmatrix}
\tag{3}
$$

The Kalman gain matrix is calculated by:

$$
\hat{K}_k = P_k^- H^T (H P_k^- H^T + R_k)^{-1}
\tag{4}
$$

where P_k^- is the "a priori" error covariance, H is the Jacobian matrix that relates the measurement to the system state vector, and R_k is the measurement noise covariance matrix. We compute P_k^- and H_k in the standard manner. The measurement noise covariance R presents the level of trust of the measurement. To enable the Kalman filter to adapt to track both normal-speed motion and abrupt motion, we divide R into two parts, normal measurement noise covariance R_a and adaptive noise covariance R_b:

$$
R = R_a + R_b
\tag{5}
$$

In our approach, we use the accelerometer to sense the gravity vector. In the ideal case, the quadratic sum of the accelerometer measurements, A_x, A_y and A_z, should be g^2, where g is gravity. But, the accelerometer reading is also affected by motion (acceleration). We therefore define our error model as the difference between the quadratic sum and g^2, as follows:

$$R_b = \left| Ax^2 + Ay^2 + Az^2 - g^2 \right| \tag{6}$$

The measurement update is:

$$\hat{X}_k = \hat{X}_k^- + \hat{K}_k(Z_k - H\hat{X}_k^-) \tag{7}$$

where the orientations are converted from quaternions to Euler angles, subtracted, and then converted back to quaternions. The measurement model for the accelerometer and magnetometer readings mentioned in [6] is used to define the system measurement Z_k.

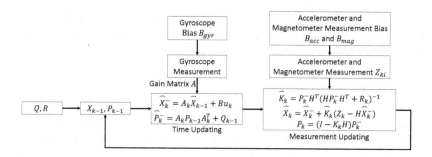

Fig. 4. Block diagram of Kalman Filter for orientation estimation

2.3   Position Estimation

When all the marker points are in the field of view, the camera can capture the position and orientation of the whole marker frame from the spatial position of the marker points. As soon as any of the marker points is blocked, the camera cannot give the orientation of the marker frame. But, it is still possible to obtain the position of any marker that is in the field of view (see Fig. 5). For the Micron Tracker, these stray markers are called XPoints. Other tracking systems, such as Polaris (Northern Digital, Inc., Waterloo, Canada) can also provide the positions of stray markers (i.e., those not associated with a defined rigid body).

But, although we can obtain the position, P_n of a stray marker, it is necessary to compute the position of the frame origin P_o. This requires three pieces of information: (1) identification of which marker point (n) was measured, (2) the distance vector (d_n) from this point to the frame origin, and (3) the orientation, R, of the reference frame, as illustrated in the following equation:

$$P_o = P_n - Rd_n \tag{8}$$

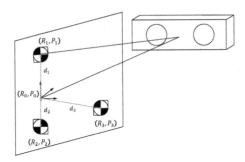

Fig. 5. When all markers are visible, the 6D pose of the reference frame, (R_0, P_0), can be calculated; if any marker is blocked, only the 3D positions, P_i, of the visible markers ($i = 1, 2,$ or 3) are available

where d_n is obtained from the marker definition file and R is obtained from the IMU measurements, as described in Section 2.2. The identification of the marker point, n, is done using a nearest neighbor approach where the position of the marker is compared to the prior estimated positions of all markers, and the closest marker selected.

3   Experiments and Results

The hybrid tracking system (IMU and camera) was mounted on a helmet and moved in random 6-D motions. All sensor data was captured by the host PC. The raw data contained valid data for all markers (i.e., there were no actual occlusions). To test the tracking performance under partial occlusion conditions, we temporarily invalidated some of the recorded marker positions. This stopped the bias estimation process and relied on the orientation estimated from the IMU measurements (Section 2.2) to recover the frame origin, as described in Section 2.3. Note that in our system, the orientation is always estimated by the IMU, so the only effect of marker occlusion is to stop estimation of the bias terms.

We sequentially rotated the tracking unit by about 40 degrees around each of the three axes. Figure 6-left shows the estimated orientation under partial occlusion conditions. As expected, there is no noticeable impact on the estimated orientation when the markers are blocked because the orientation is computed from the inertial sensor data. Thus, the only effect of marker occlusion is that sensor biases are not compensated by the optical tracking data. To determine the typical drift rates for the inertial sensor biases, we performed an experiment where we computed the orientation from the inertial data over a 24 minute time interval, with a stationary sensor. We expressed the orientation as pitch, roll, and yaw angles, and computed the RMS errors by first subtracting the mean value from each set of angles. The resulting RMS orientation errors, expressed as pitch, roll, and yaw, were 0.0821, 0.0495, and 0.0917 degrees, respectively. This data characterized the orientation error due to both sensor bias drift and noise (Fig. 7).

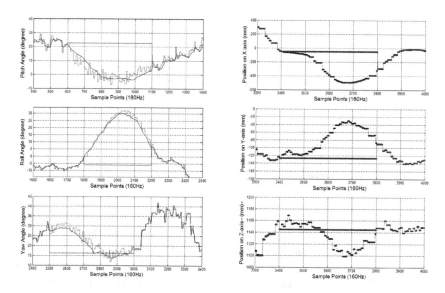

Fig. 6. Left: Orientation estimated by optical tracker (blue line) and our proposed method (black line), when we simulate partial occlusion for sample points 600-1000, 1800-2200 and 2500-3000. Red line shows the ground-truth, which is provided by the optical tracker. Right: Position estimated by optical tracker (blue line) and our proposed method (black line), when we simulate partial occlusion for sample points 3400-3800. Red line shows the ground-truth position from the optical tracker.

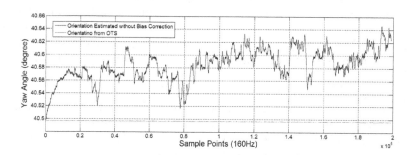

Fig. 7. Yaw angle measured by optical tracker (red) and IMU without bias correction (blue) over a 24 minute interval

We then performed experiments to demonstrate the estimation of the position under partial occlusion conditions. We manually moved the hybrid tracking system in the X, Y, and Z directions, as shown in Fig. 6-right. The position error due to partial occlusion is relatively small, even though it is affected by inaccuracies in both the position and orientation measurements. This is illustrated in Fig. 8, which shows the difference between the frame origin reported by the Micron Tracker (since it was never really blocked) and the position estimated by our method, with simulated blocking of all but one marker.

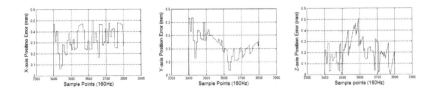

Fig. 8. Position errors for the three axes during simulated occlusion of all but one marker

4   Conclusions and Future Work

This paper presented a sensor fusion approach that uses inertial measurements to compensate for partial occlusion of optically-tracked markers. In contrast to other approaches, the orientation is always obtained from the inertial measurements, via a Kalman Filter where the system dynamics are driven by the gyroscope and the accelerometer and magnetometer provide measurement updates. Rather than discarding the orientation measured by the camera, however, we use it to estimate the bias of the inertial sensors (gyroscope, accelerometer, and magnetometer). The position is always obtained from the optical tracker, because we assume that at least one marker will be visible. If some markers are occluded, however, the optical tracker can only provide the positions of the visible markers and therefore we use the marker design geometry, in conjunction with the IMU-estimated orientation, to compute the frame position.

In practice, we expect that this sensor fusion approach will provide good accuracy over relatively long periods of partial marker occlusion. The determining factors include the stability of the estimated bias terms. If the sensor biases drift, it will be necessary to restore full line-of-sight so that the biases can be re-estimated. This is particularly important for the magnetometer bias, which can have large variations due to magnetic field disturbances.

Our experimental results showed good accuracy during the partial occlusion cases, but further improvements are possible. First, we can compensate for the small time difference between the optical tracker and IMU measurements. Second, we can better estimate the gravity vector in the presence of body accelerations, as done in our prior work that used a Kalman Filter to estimate the gravity from the "noisy" accelerometer measurements [7]. Another possibility is to estimate the acceleration from the optical tracker positions. Third, we currently compute the gyroscope bias by numerically differentiating the orientation angles measured by the camera; it would likely be better to use a Kalman Filter. We could also estimate the gyroscope bias in the orientation EKF, as in [11][7]. Fourth, our current implementation uses just a single visible marker in the partial occlusion case, but the method can be extended to use all visible markers. Finally, the results reported here relied on offline processing of the sensor data. We are currently implementing a real-time version in C++ to support online testing of the hybrid tracking system with augmented reality overlays.

Acknowledgements. We thank Jayfus Doswell and Juxtopia LLC for providing the optical see-through goggles and Dr. George Jallo for his clinical guidance. Dr. Kaisorn Chaichana performed the cadaver experiments. Changyu He received support from the Chinese Scholarship Council. Praneeth Sadda was supported by a JHU Provost Undergraduate Research Award (PURA).

References

1. Azimi, E., Doswell, J., Kazanzides, P.: Augmented reality goggles with an integrated tracking system for navigation in neurosurgery. In: Proc. IEEE Virtual Reality, Orange County, CA, pp. 123–124 (March 2012)
2. Azuma, R., Bishop, G.: Improving static and dynamic registration in an optical see-through HMD. In: SIGGRAPH, pp. 197–204 (July 1994)
3. Chai, L., Hoff, W.A., Vincent, T.: Three-dimensional motion and structure estimation using inertial sensors and computer vision for augmented reality. Presence 11(5), 474–492 (2002)
4. Hoff, W., Vincent, T.: Analysis of head pose accuracy in augmented reality. IEEE Trans. Visualization and Computer Graphics 6(4), 319–334 (2000)
5. Park, F.C., Martin, B.J.: Robot sensor calibration: Solving AX = XB on the Euclidean group. IEEE Trans. on Robotics and Auto. 10(5), 717–721 (1994)
6. Ren, H., Kazanzides, P.: Hybrid attitude estimation for laparoscopic surgical tools: A preliminary study. In: Intl. Conf. of IEEE Engineering in Medicine and Biology Society (EMBC), pp. 5583–5586 (September 2009)
7. Ren, H., Kazanzides, P.: Investigation of attitude tracking using an integrated inertial and magnetic navigation system for hand-held surgical instruments. IEEE/ASME Trans. on Mechatronics 17(2), 210–217 (2012)
8. Sadda, P., Azimi, E., Jallo, G., Doswell, J., Kazanzides, P.: Surgical navigation with a head-mounted tracking system and display. Medicine Meets Virtual Reality (MMVR) 20, 363–369 (2013)
9. Sauer, F., Wenzel, F., Vogt, S., Tao, Y., Genc, Y., Bani-Hashemi, A.: Augmented workspace: designing an AR testbed. In: Proc. IEEE Intl. Symp. on Augmented Reality (ISAR), pp. 47–53 (October 2000)
10. Tao, Y., Hu, H., Zhou, H.: Integration of vision and inertial sensors for 3D arm motion tracking in home-based rehabilitation. Intl. J. of Robotics Research 26(6), 607–624 (2007)
11. Tobergte, A., Pomarlan, M., Hirzinger, G.: Robust multi sensor pose estimation for medical applications. In: Proc. IEEE/RSJ Intl. Conf. on Intell, St. Louis, MO, pp. 492–497 (October 2009)
12. Vaccarella, A., De Momi, E., Enquobahrie, A., Ferrigno, G.: Unscented Kalman filter based sensor fusion for robust optical and electromagnetic tracking in surgical navigation. IEEE/ASME Trans. on Instrumentation and Measurement 62(7), 2067–2081 (2013)
13. You, S., Neumann, U., Azuma, R.: Hybrid inertial and vision tracking for augmented reality registration. In: Proc. IEEE Conf. on Virtual Reality, Houston, TX, pp. 260–267 (March 1999)

Improvement of a Virtual Pivot
for Minimally Invasive Surgery Simulators
Using Haptic Augmentation

Mohammad F. Obeid[1], Salim Chemlal[2], Krzysztof J. Rechowicz[3],
Eun-sil Heo[1], Robert E. Kelly[4], and Frederic D. McKenzie[1,*]

[1] Dept. of Modeling, Simulation, and Visualization Engineering,
Old Dominion University, Norfolk, USA
{mobei001,eheox002,rdmckenz}@odu.edu
[2] Dept. of Electrical and Computer Engineering,
Old Dominion University, Norfolk, USA
schem001@odu.edu
[3] Virginia Modeling, Analysis and Simulation Center,
Old Dominion University, Norfolk, USA
krechowi@odu.edu
[4] Pediatric Surgery, Children's Hospital of The King's Daughters
and Eastern Virginia Medical School, Norfolk, USA
robert.kelly@chkd.org

Abstract. With rapid development of minimally invasive surgery, proficiency with intricate skills is becoming a greater concern. Consequently, the use of out-of-operating room training has increased significantly through employing high-fidelity and anatomically-correct graphics and haptic interfaces in virtual reality simulations. The effort in developing surgical simulators for generic minimally invasive procedures is still, however, suboptimal for many haptic implementations. A main aspect of such simulations is the pivoting behavior of the surgical tool realized using the haptic device. This paper investigates the limitation of a fully-virtual implementation of the pivot and the ability to augment haptic interfaces to achieve a natural representation of forces. The design and implementation of two surgical tool pivoting techniques are introduced. Furthermore, a phantom is constructed from synthesized components to be used to measure and reproduce realistic mechanical properties of the anatomical model and pivot behavior.

Keywords: Haptic augmented reality, Surgical simulation, Hybrid simulation.

1 Introduction

For the majority of the 20th century surgeons opted for open surgery, which usually contradicts patients' desire to have the least invasive procedure possible. The need for minimally invasive procedures is not only related to excessive

---

* Corresponding author.

C.A. Linte et al. (Eds.): AE-CAI 2014, LNCS 8678, pp. 70–79, 2014.

scaring but also to iatrogenic damage caused while achieving the goal of the surgery. The benefits posed by Minimally Invasive Procedures (MIP), such as decreased mortality rates, faster recoveries, shorter hospital stays, as well as minimal scaring and pain, changed the medical community's view on such procedures. Advancements in external imaging have also significantly contributed to a wider use of MIP over exploratory surgery [3].

In order to explore this topic, it is necessary to first define minimally invasive surgery. Laparoscopic surgery is often mistakenly considered a synonym of MIP. It is worth pointing out, however, that a MIP can be defined as any medical procedure that is less invasive than an equivalent open surgery alternative for the same purpose. A great example of a non-laparoscopic MIP is the Nuss procedure, also called Minimally Invasive Repair of Pectus Excavatum (MIRPE), which is an alternative to the Ravtich procedure and involves inserting a concave stainless steel bar posterior to the sternum and anterior to the pericardium, monitored by a thoracoscope. The Ravitch procedure is an open surgery technique which requires a long incision along the chest; whereas the Nuss procedure requires only two relatively small incisions on either sides of the chest. Although the Nuss procedure is more invasive than a typical laparoscopic surgery, it is significantly less invasive than its open surgery alternative.

Despite all advantages of MIP, however, the procedure may be more challenging from the surgeon's perspective than open surgery, usually because of the limited room for motion and decreased dexterity. In addition, since interaction with tissues is via instruments and graspers rather than direct manipulation, a surgeon's depth perception may be negatively affected which can impair judgment on how much force to apply; thus introducing risks of complications. Furthermore, since the tool rotates around the pivot, the endpoint moves in the opposite direction to the surgeon's hands, making required motor skills difficult to learn [6].

Training and proper surgical planning can alleviate the limitations of MIPs. There is a number of commercially available and under development simulators for MIPs for the most common laparoscopic procedures; including cases from general surgery, gynecology, bariatric and colon surgery. To fully leverage benefits of surgical simulation, interaction with the training environment should be performed with 3D user interfaces (3D UI) modeled to accurately mimic surgical instrumentation including tactile feedback. Several approaches for achieving this goal can be identified. Bachofen et al. [1] modified the actual surgical instrument to allow natural control of the surgical procedure and force feedback in hysteroscopy simulation. Baur et al. [2] implemented a novel haptic interface taking into account constraints of endoscopic surgery. Several companies offer haptic devices for specific medical procedures. Mentice (Gothenburg, Sweden) [8], the first manufacturer of the simulation system for laparoscopic procedures, markets two lines of specialized medical force feedback interfaces for the emulation of endoscopic instruments and for the simulation of interventional procedures including interventional radiology.

Some simulators introduce actual minimally invasive instrumentation through physical ports which are typically located on an arbitrary object like a box or hemisphere [11] or on an anatomically correct phantom [7]. Another approach is to augment commercial force feedback devices. Coles et al. [5] replaced the standard end effector of a Geomagic Omni haptic device, used in needle insertion simulation - PalpSim, with a real needle hub and shortened needle shaft. The same off-the-shelf commercial haptic devices were used by Sankaranarayanan et al. [10] as the base for their laparoscopic adjustable gastric band simulator. The actual laparoscopic tools were attached in place of the end effector.

Challenges arise when a non-laparoscopic MIP is to be simulated. Using the Nuss procedure as an example, the surgical tool, called an introducer, is curved and, depending on the stage of the procedure, can move freely in space or could be in collision. From the 3D user interface perspective, it can be problematic to simulate all phenomena occurring during the procedure unless performed in stages, using different setups to accommodate each stage of the surgery. Since such intermittent simulation techniques may be impractical and don't promise delivering the required surgical skills, in this work we propose a methodology to simulate pivoting mechanisms for general MIPs using generic haptic interfaces and low cost rapid prototyping techniques.

2   Methods

Many surgical simulators that incorporate haptic interfaces use physical components when simulating an insertion, i.e. pivot, point for the tool; whereas others utilize haptic feedback to achieve this purpose. Depending on the nature of the procedure, a physical constituent can be of great significance to enhance realism aspects. This section describes the methods used to construct both virtual and hybrid (augmented) pivots for minimally invasive procedures to show how one can better the other. The hybrid description here denotes an augmented reality design based on touch augmentation.

2.1   Virtual Pivot

In any MIP, the surgical tool's movement is limited at the insertion point and by the room for motion inside the body. These constraints can be simulated by applying various forces that vary depending on the stiffness of the tissue or surrounding organs.

As explained in more detail in [4], the pivoting behavior of the tool at the insertion point can be approximated using a fully-virtual setup utilizing forces from the haptic device; the haptic device acts as a virtual pivot constraining the tool from motion in the local x- and y-directions by applying high stiffness forces while allowing translation in the z-direction only. The z-direction motion is along the axis of the tool at the point of the pivot allowing further insertion. This absence of force in the z-direction is altered depending on the orientation of the haptic device's stylus, i.e., the movement is allowed in the local z-direction of the stylus which is reoriented in real-time when the stylus is rotated. Light friction force is applied in the local z-direction when moving through the pivot to simulate friction generated between the tool and the skin at the insertion area. In order to apply such accurate forces in all the corresponding haptic device local axes, global force components are to constantly be converted to local force components, as described below:

1. Get current rotation matrix R.
2. Get total displacement vector, d, between initial and current positions.
3. Multiply R by d to get the local translation vector t_L.
4. Multiply t_L by the scaling vector $< 1, 1, 0 >$ to get new local translation vector t_{LS}.
5. Multiply inverse of rotation matrix, R^{-1}, by t_{LS} to get force components in the local coordinates of the haptic device.

Although the force models for constraining the haptic device's motion and for simulating collisions are a successful approximation of the tool's pivoting behavior, the approach itself has a serious limitation. Since the user is able to move the stylus in and out (or forward/backward) at the insertion point, the end effector is always carried along causing the stylus' physical joint to be located, at some instances, at coordinates that correspond to the inside of the patient. In addition, since a 3-degrees of freedom (DOF) force feedback device is unable to provide rotational forces at the end effector, collisions resulting from rotational motions cannot be directly represented.

2.2 Hybrid Pivot

Given the nature of generic (3-DOF) haptic device's end effector, no insertion mechanism can be performed without carrying the stylus' natural pivot along, i.e., the stylus joint will physically travel with the tool inside the object's co-ordinates whereas, in reality, the tool is inserted inside while its pivot is at the insertion point. This discrepancy will, therefore, have to be compensated for by augmenting the generic haptic device with an extension that implements a mechanism to utilize the device's natural pivot, while allowing the tool to move appropriately.

After performing the necessary measurements of the haptic device's stylus and associated components, this mechanism was designed, 3D-modeled, and proto-typed using 3D printing (MakerBot Replicator 2X). The mechanism is composed of two main components: a translation component that controls and monitors the translational motion of the tool; and a force feedback component which produces haptic force feedback upon collision. The mechanism is controlled by the Arduino Uno - a low cost open-source prototyping platform. This extension is mounted onto the stylus and travels with it in all directions before insertion.

At insertion, force is applied from the haptic device to prevent motion in all directions. As the user attempts to move the tool through the insertion point (in the z-direction), the tool – not the stylus itself – slides through the extension affecting, and affected by, two rubber wheels located on top of and below the tool (Figure 1a). To replicate translational movement with respect to the fixed pivot, the tool's motion will rotate the lower wheel affecting a rotary encoder (potentiometer), the rotation of which is converted into translation of the surgical tool in the simulation. At any instance, if the surgical tool collides with an organ in the simulation, e.g. the pericardium in the case of the Nuss procedure, a signal will be sent to Arduino to actuate a motor within the extension's assembly that rotates a spirally threaded beam. As a result of the beam's rotation, the axis holding the second, upper, wheel will descend vertically pushing it onto the tool; thus reproducing force that would hinder the tool's motion (Figure 1b).

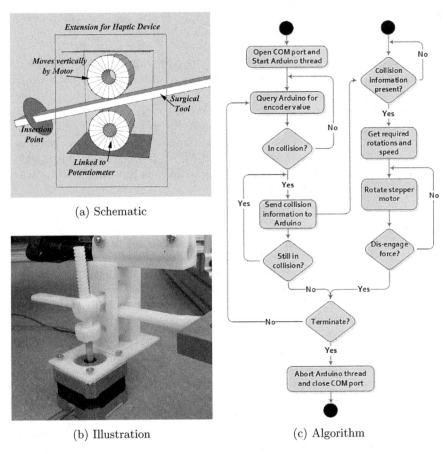

(a) Schematic   (b) Illustration   (c) Algorithm

Fig. 1. Hybrid pivot mechanism for the haptic device augmentation: (a) a schematic showing the components of the extension's assembly, (b) an illustration of the actual assembly, and (c) the algorithm for information querying and command execution

A driver for the haptic device's extension was implemented in Unity. The simulation engine queries the encoder's reading and sends collision information to Arduino asynchronously due to different update rates. For the same reason, the motor is controlled asynchronously so that encoder information can be acquired even when the motor is executing the previously assigned command (Figure 1c).

Implementing this mechanism by adding this extension to the device's end effector facilitates simulating an insertion behavior where the end effector is constrained from moving, while the user can maneuver through the extension utilizing the stylus' natural pivot, thus resolving the previously described discrepancy.

3   Case Study: The Nuss Procedure Surgical Simulator

The Nuss procedure is a minimally invasive technique for repairing pectus excavatum (PE) (a congenital chest wall deformity occurring primarily in children and young adults). In this procedure, the surgeon uses a surgical tool (introducer) to make a pathway through the mediastinum, under the sternum and anterior to the pericardium. A pre-bent steel bar is then pulled through the pathway and flipped to elevate the sternum's position and is sutured and secured into place. The bar is removed after a period of two to three years producing a significant and permanent improvement in the shape of the chest.

As described in [9], the Nuss Procedure Surgical Simulator (NPSS) was developed to provide a training platform for this procedure. The simulator setup integrates an external and an internal (thoracoscopic) view of the patient in the virtual environment, with incorporation of a haptic interface used for moving the surgical tool in the scene.

As discussed in previous sections, to faithfully represent the surgical tool's behavior at the insertion point into the chest, a hybrid pivoting mechanism was developed. However, to be able to quantify the forces exerted in the simulation, an experimental platform is necessary to be used as a representation of the real system.

3.1   Phantom Design

In order to generate realistic displacement and force values to be used in the simulation, a physical phantom was constructed. This phantom incorporates the use of the haptic device to measure real-time displacement, a load cell to measure real-time forces, and a synthetic tissue to represent an organ in the thoracic cavity. The haptic device used is a 3-DOF Geomagic Phantom Premium 1.5 high force feedback device. The load cell used is a National Instruments Omega High Accuracy S Beam with 250 lbs capacity and 25 kHz measuring frequency. The load cell was fitted onto the 3D printed tool to measure compression force, and the haptic device's end effector was mounted onto the tool from the other side.

Using LabView, real-time continuous displacement and force values were collected and synchronized. Position was tracked using an integrated dynamic-link library for the haptic device and forces were collected from the load cell's physical channel. Since the load cell and the haptic device operate at different frequencies, the lower frequency of both, 1 kHz, was standardized when querying the values.

3.2   Implementation and Results

The phantom constructed was used to collect mechanical properties of the synthetic tissue. System damping was first measured without colliding with the synthetic tissue. Results showed that for velocity between 0 and 1.5 mm/s, damping force increases linearly; and between 1.5 and 7 mm/s it is equal to 0.8 N. The combination of this information with the force-displacement data collected from collision with the synthetic tissue suggested modeling the spring coefficient as a nonlinear element. The force model can be represented by:

$$F(x) = \begin{cases} a_1 x^2 + a_2 x + a_3 - b_1 \dot{x} - b_2 & \text{, if in collision} \\ -b_1 \dot{x} - b_2 & \text{, otherwise} \end{cases} \tag{1}$$

where a_k are coefficients of the 2nd order polynomial corresponding to the spring component and b_l are coefficients corresponding to the damping component.

After constructing the force model and obtaining the required material properties, the simulation model was calibrated to reflect a similar behavior. Using the known measurements of the haptic device's extension assembly, the amount of force exerted by the wheel on the tool as a result of the motor's motion can be quantified. One full rotation of the motor's beam will cause the rubber wheel to descend two millimeters vertically squeezing the tool. It was observed that one millimeter of vertical motion will add 0.2 N force hindering the tool's motion.

Since damping is inherently present in the mechanism, simply positioning the wheel to exert the right amount of friction force will suffice, whereas collision force was simulated by complementing the program with the force model.

3.3   Validation Experiment

To add more realism to the user interface, a handle for the surgical tool (introducer) was reproduced to scale and was integrated with the haptic device's extension. In addition, an object was modeled and prototyped to replicate half a torso and was covered with synthetic skin; where the user is able to make an incision at the insertion point (Figure 2).

In order to investigate the faithfulness of the simulation after integrating the measured properties, the load cell was integrated on the tool as it slides through the hybrid pivot to measure real-time force applied by the wheel; and the rotary encoder that controls the position of the simulated tool was used to record real-time displacement (Figure 2). The measured and simulated results were compared as depicted in Figure 3. As observed in Figure 3, the difference between the measured and simulated force-displacement profiles is not greater than 0.05 N in general. When displacement approaches 15 mm, the difference increases to 0.15 N. Slight instability of the simulated force comes from inertia of the system. The results show that the simulation was able to approximate the behavior observed on the phantom.

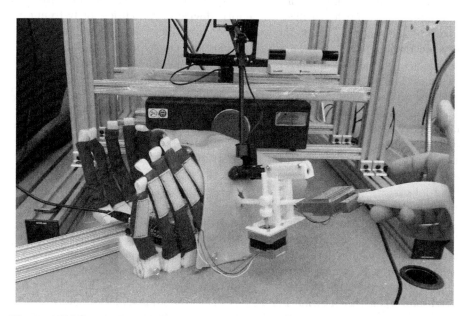

Fig. 2. NPSS setup with hybrid pivot implemented, illustrating the incorporation of the load cell for real-time force gauge

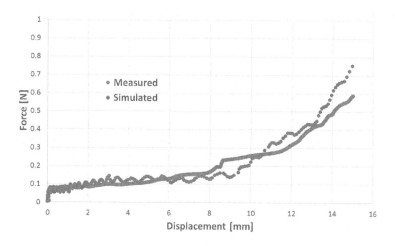

Fig. 3. Comparison of measured and simulated force-displacement profiles

4 Conclusion

In this paper, two techniques for implementing a surgical tool's pivoting behavior in a surgical simulation environment were discussed. The first one is a fully virtual implementation that utilizes the haptic device's capabilities solely to apply force when necessary. This method, however, introduced a position discrepancy between the simulated and the physical (natural) pivot of the tool. The second technique introduces a supplemental component that can be mounted on generic haptic devices to augment the exerted forces and implement a hybrid pivoting mechanism. This component doesn't require a physical port to constrain the tool's motion in space as that can be achieved using forces applied from the haptic device; but nonetheless, an anatomically correct object can be used to increase realism and achieve higher forces needed by other aspects of the procedure. As the tool is moved into the insertion point, the natural pivot of the device's end effector stays fixed while the tool slides through the mechanism. The tool's position is tracked in real-time and force is applied to it according to corresponding collisions from the virtual environment.

The mechanism was validated using a constructed phantom representing a patient's internal organs and was able to provide accurate force and displacement profiles. Information regarding the force's behavior over time or versus displacement and velocity is now directly obtainable. This instrumented tool can be utilized to describe the mechanical properties of any object and is, therefore, very useful to extract information as part of testing and validation efforts.

Future work includes the use of the phantom to measure force properties from cadavers and/or real patients instead of synthetic tissue to provide realistic description of forces. The hybrid pivot can be improved to include stronger motors that can represent collisions with rigid anatomies such as bones. Furthermore, a 6-DOF haptic device will supplement the current setup to incorporate torque force feedback upon rotating the tool around the pivot.

References

1. Bachofen, D., Zatonyi, J., Harders, M., Szekely, G., Fruh, P., Thaler, M.: Enhancing the visual realism of hysteroscopy simulation. In: Medicine Meets Virtual Reality 14, vol. 119, pp. 31–36 (2006)
2. Baur, C., Guzzoni, D., Georg, O.: Virgy: a virtual reality and force feedback based endoscopic surgery simulator. Studies in Health Technology and Informatics 50, 110–116 (1998)
3. Biere, S.S., Cuesta, M.A., van der Peet, D.L.: Minimally invasive versus open esophagectomy for cancer: a systematic review and meta-analysis. Minerva Chirurgica 64(2), 121–133 (2009)
4. Chemlal, S., Rechowicz, K.J., Obeid, M.F., Kelly, R.E., McKenzie, F.D.: Developing clinically relevant aspects of the nuss procedure surgical simulator. In: Medicine Meets Virtual Reality 21, vol. 196, pp. 51–55 (2014)
5. Coles, T., John, N., Sofia, G., Gould, D., Caldwell, D.: Modification of commercial force feedback hardware for needle insertion simulation. Studies in Health Technology and Informatics 163, 135–137 (2011)

6. Gallagher, A.G., McClure, N., McGuigan, J., Ritchie, K., Sheehy, N.P.: An ergonomic analysis of the fulcrum effect in the acquisition of endoscopic skills. Endoscopy 30(7), 617–620 (1998)
7. Laedral: Virtual i.v. simulator,
   www.laerdal.com/us/doc/245/Virtual-I-V--Simulator
8. Mentice: Medical simulator, www.mentice.com
9. Rechowicz, K.J., Obeid, M.F., Chemlal, S., McKenzie, F.D.: Simulation of the critical steps of the nuss procedure. Computer Methods in Biomechanics and Biomedical Engineering: Imaging & Visualization 2, 1–15 (2014)
10. Sankaranarayanan, G., Adair, J., Halic, T., Gromski, M., Lu, Z., Ahn, W., Jones, D., De, S.: Validation of a novel laparoscopic adjustable gastric band simulator. Surgical Endoscopy 25(4), 1012–1018 (2011)
11. SimSurgery: Sep - surgical simulation platform, www.simsurgery.com

Augmented Reality in Neurovascular Surgery: First Experiences

Marta Kersten-Oertel, Ian Gerard, Simon Drouin, Kelvin Mok,
Denis Sirhan, David Sinclair, and D. Louis Collins

Montreal Neurological Institute & Hospital, McGill University, Montreal, Canada

Abstract. In neurovascular surgery, the surgeon must navigate among eloquent areas, through complex neurovascular anatomy to a particular vascular malformation or anomaly. Augmented reality (AR) visualization may be used to show vessels not visible when looking at the brain surface and to aid navigation by bringing into spatial alignment pre-operative vascular data with the real patient anatomy. In using AR, we may aid the surgeon in planning the craniotomy to obtain the optimal resection corridor and reduce the time to localize and identify important vessels. In the following paper, we describe the first uses of our AR neuronavigation system in the operating room (OR). Specifically, we describe the system's use in three different neurovascular cases, an aneurysm case, an arteriovenous malfromation, and a dural arteriovenous fistula. Furthermore, we give a qualitative evaluation based on comments from the OR and post-operative discussions with the neurosurgeons.

1 Introduction

Augmented reality visualizations are being increasingly studied in the domain of image-guided surgery (IGS). In augmented reality (AR) IGS, virtual images of patient anatomy and/or physiology are overlaid onto the real anatomy of the patient giving the surgeon both contextual anatomical information and specific enhanced information about the location of regions of interest. AR IGS systems have the potential to (1) decrease the cognitive workload of the surgeon by bringing into spatial alignment pre-operative patient images with the pertinent anatomy of the patient in the operating room (OR) and (2) to improve patient outcomes by allowing for improved intra-operative planning, guidance and navigation. Yet, to date very few of the proposed AR IGS systems have been used by surgeons in the OR. In a recent review of mixed reality image-guided surgery (IGS) systems it was shown that only one third of the proposed mixed reality IGS systems reviewed were evaluated in terms of their overall use in the OR or the feasibility of bringing the system within the OR [6].

In this paper, we give a description of the first experiences of our AR IGS system applied to neurovascular surgery. In particular, we describe the first use of our system in three surgical cases for neurovascular surgery: an aneurysm case, an arteriovenous malformation (AVM), and a dural arteriovenous fistula. We describe not only the positive results and the feedback from the neurosurgeons

C.A. Linte et al. (Eds.): AE-CAI 2014, LNCS 8678, pp. 80–89, 2014.

who used the system but also some of the pitfalls encountered and how they have shaped, and are shaping, the continued development of our AR image-guided neurosurgery (IGNS) system.

2   Background

A number of systems have been proposed for AR image-guided neurosurgery, for example the MAGI system by Edwards *et al.* [4], Birkfellner *et al's* Variscope AR [1], and Paul *et al.* mixed reality system for IGNS [9]. In a recent and related paper, Cabrilo *et al.* [2] described the use of one of the only commercial AR systems for neuronavigation, the Zeiss Pentero 900 (Zeiss, Oberkochen, Germany) neurosurgical microscope. The system was used for surgery in 28 aneurysm cases. The segmented aneurysms and nearby vessels were projected into one of the oculars of the microscope. Based on their study, the authors concluded that AR may add to the minimally invasiveness of the surgery but that more studies are needed and better techniques need to be developed to improve user-friendliness. Of note in this system, is the need for better visualization techniques which would help in the depth perception of the vessels and aneurysms (which appear to be floating above the brain surface). For a more thorough review of AR in IGNS, and IGS in general, the reader is referred to [6].

3   AR IGNS System

The developed system and its main components have been previously described in [3,8]. Here, the major components (relevant to the three clinical cases for which it was used) are summarized using the DVV (Data, Visualization processing, View) taxonomy [7].

3.1   Data

The current main application of the described AR IGNS system is neurovascular surgery, therefore, the imaging datasets that we use are digital subtraction computed tomography angiography (DS CTA). Vessels are extracted from the DS CTA using thresholding and volume rendered on the navigation system.

3.2   Visualization Processing

A number of different volume rendering techniques, including chromadepth, fog, stereopsis, and colour coding have been explored for enhanced depth perception and visualization of neurovasculature [5]. In the three clinical cases in which the system was used we explored depicting edges and colour-coding.

The volume rendered virtual vessels obtained from DS CTA are merged with the live camera image using alpha blending. In particular we modulate the opacity of the camera image to show more of the virtual volume rendered object in the region of the surgical target and more of the camera image elsewhere. In order to display the virtual vasculature to look like it is within the brain rather than floating above the brain we use the cue of occlusion. This is achieved by extracting edges from the camera image in the area where the image is more transparent. To find those edges we use an OpenGL fragment shader that computes an approximation of the gradient of the image using a Sobel filter. The resolution of the live camera image is 640x480 and images are augmented at 30 frames/second. Details of our method are given in [8].

3.3   View

For *display* we use the monitor of our neuronavigation system, making the *perception location* of the augmented reality visualization the digital monitor. In order to capture images of the live patient a tracked video camera, Sony HDR-XR150, was used. The video camera was outfitted with an infra-red tracker as can be seen in Fig. 1, left.

In terms of interactions, the surgeon does not directly interact with the system, rather the developers/technicians work the navigation system. All of the visualization parameters can all be changed on the fly, e.g. fog can be turned on and off, edge detection of the camera image can be turned on and off, and the transfer functions which affect the volume rendering can also be changed.

4   Methods

The aim of this work was to use and qualitatively evaluate our AR IGNS system with surgeons in the OR during real surgical cases. To this end, our system was brought into the OR for three cases, described below.[1] During all three cases the system was used at several points during the surgery. The proposed AR system was used in parallel with the commercial neuronavigation system (Medtronic Stealthstation, Medtronic Inc.). Patient-to-image landmark registration was done simultaneously on both systems, to reduce redundancy and extra work in the OR.

The calibrated and tracked video camera described in the previous section was used to capture live images of the patients' anatomy. The camera was handled by a surgeon who was not scrubbed in at the time and was able to handle the camera near to the patient without disturbing the sterile field. Our set-up in the OR is shown in Fig 1. The system was used by two neurosurgeons from the Montreal Neurological Institute, Montreal, Quebec, Canada, specializing in neurovascular surgery. One surgeon performed the first and second case and a second neurosurgeon used the system in the third case.

For all cases the camera calibration error (misalignment between virtual and real patient) was 2.1 mm and the initial patient-to-image registration fiducial registration error (FRE) was between 2.6 mm and 4.2 mm. Resulting in a reasonable registration between the real patient and overlaid virtual images.

---

[1] Ethics approval for this project was obtained from the Research and Ethics Board at the Montreal Neurological Institute.

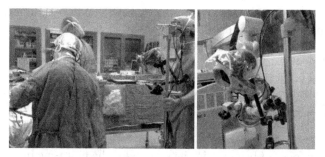

Fig. 1. The tracked camera was attached to an IV pole and used at a number of different points during the surgery

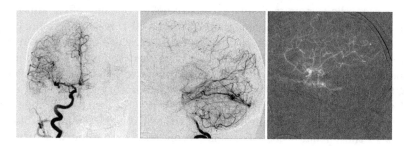

Fig. 2. Cerebral X–ray angiography images indicating: *Left:* one aneurysm on inferior division of MCA (pink arrow) and second aneurysm at A1/ACOM junction (blue arrow) *Center:* a left inferior temporal AVM (pink arrow) and *Right:* a type II Borden dural AV fistula, post embolization, (pink arrow). Note that these images were used for diagnosis and not navigation.

5   Surgical Cases

The proposed AR neuronavigation system was brought into the OR for three neurovascular surgeries: an aneurysm, an arteriovenous malformation, and an arteriovenous fisula. Diagnostic X-ray angiography images with each of the anomalies/malformations indicated within the image are shown in Fig 2.

During all three cases we were able to successfully register the patient to the pre-operative data, track the surgical probe and display an AR view with virtual pre-operative images aligned to the patient's real anatomy. When the video camera was not used, our system provided standard neuronavigation information (i.e. the location of a tracked surgical probe with respect to the pre-operative patient anatomy). Our experiences for each case are described below.

5.1   Case 1: Aneurysm

Aneurisms are localized blood-filled balloon-like swellings arising from the wall of a blood vessel. As an aneurysm increases in size its wall weakens and there is an increased risk of rupture. There are two common treatment options for cerebral aneurysms: (1) surgical clipping, and (2) endovascular coiling. With surgical clipping, a strong metallic clip is placed at the base, or neck of the aneurysm in order to exclude the aneurism from the circulation.

The developed system was first used in the OR for a craniotomy to clip two aneurisms in a 52 year old female (where endovascular treatment was not feasible). One multilobed aneurysm was at the bifurcation of the middle cerebral artery (MCA), involving mainly the inferior division of the MCA. The second was a ruptured anterior communicating multilobed aneurysm at an unusually fenestrated A1/ACOM junction (Fig 2 left).

The primary focus of bringing in the system for the first time into the OR was to determine how to efficiently incorporate the research system into the surgical workflow and to determine how and when it could be used during surgery. During this first case, the system was only used only before opening of the dura, after which the neurosurgical microscope was brought in. At this point no more images were taken as it would have meant moving the microscope out of the way.

For this case, the vessels from the DS CTA were volume rendered in red and merged with the camera view. We found, however, that the visualizations did not perform as they had within our ideal laboratory setting. Due to the blood and numerous specular highlights caused by the bright OR lights, the Sobel filter extracted too many edges from the live camera images, blocking the view of the virtual object. For this reason, edge extraction was turned off and the virtual vessels within a defined area of interest were displayed on a grey background and outside this area the camera image was displayed (Fig 3 right). The lack of edges and depth cues made it difficult to determine the depth at which particular vessels lay and all the vessels seemed to lie within one plane. Furthermore, the vessels did not look like they were within the patient's head. Finally, since the augmented images were on the dura rather than the cortex, difficulty in interpreting vessel location was increased.

5.2   Case 2: AVM

Arteriovenous malformations (AVMs) are abnormal collections of blood vessels. The main constituents or nidus of an AVM are abnormal vessels that are hybrids between true arteries and veins. AVMs are fed by one or more arteries (feeders), and are drained by one or more major draining veins (drainers). These feeding and draining vessels often have weakened walls that may leak or rupture. The feeding and draining vessels may also be unusually large and tortuous in their course due to the abnormally high pressures and blood flow within AVMs. Surgery for AVMs is complex and involves a careful stepwise approach to identifying and isolating the margins of the malformation and then obliterating the feeding vessels and draining veins in order to safely remove the nidus. Real time intra-operative localization and identification of arteries and veins of an AVM - particularly the deeper feeding arteries is often very difficult and time consuming. These important aspects of AVM surgery can be facilitated using AR.

Our AR system was brought into a case for an AVM in a 41 year old female. Due to significant vasospasm of the left internal and left vertebral arteries,

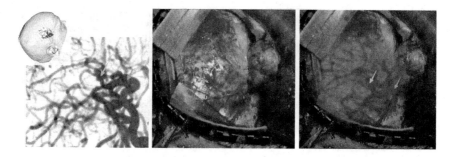

Fig. 3. *Left:* A zoomed in view of an arterial phase DS CTA howing one aneurysm on inferior division of MCA (indicated with a green arrow) and second aneurysm at A1/ACOM junction (indicated with a blue arrow). In the upper left corner we see the positioning of the patient head on the OR table and the area of the craniotomy. *Center:* Image from tracked video camera of the dura. *Right:* Augmented reality view with camera image overlaid on volume rendered red vessels (grey background). The aneurysm on inferior division of the MCA is indicated with the green arrow and the aneurysm at A1/ACOM junction is indicated with the blue arrow.

embolization was not possible and therefore, the patient underwent surgery. This was a left inferior temporal AVM fed by the inferior temporal branch of the left posterior cerebral arteries and drained via a unique cortical vein running along the inferior aspect of the temporal lobe.

Before going into the second case, we improved our edge extraction algorithm so that it would better deal with the strong OR surgical lights. To reduce the amount of edges found we first blur the camera image and then extract edges on the blurred image using a Sobel filter. This is done using a two-pass GLSL (OpenGL Shading Language)[2] fragment shader. Furthermore, we can adjust blurring in real-time to add or remove the amount of detected edges.

During the second case the surgeon commented on the ease of the initial set up of the system, and in particular the fact that the landmark patient-to-image registration is done at the same time and using the same points as the commercial system. In terms of the visualization, the surgeon was pleased with the ability to localize vessels and areas of interest that are not visible on the surface (see Fig 4). At the same time, the surgeon said that he would have liked to have not only the information about the location of a vessel but also the absolute depth of the vessel below the surface. This is something we are considering for future work.

5.3   Case 3: Fistula

An *arteriovenous (AV) dural fistula* is similar in its pathology of abnormal arterial and venous connections to that of a pial AVM but the locale is quite different. AV dural fistulas are found solely within the layers of the dura. Although the

---

[2] http://www.opengl.org/documentation/glsl/

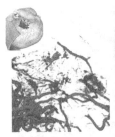 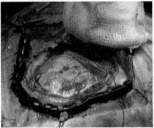 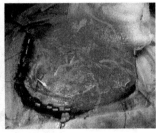

Fig. 4. *Left:* Volume rendered vessels extracted from a late phase (venous) DS CTA. The green dot on the left side indicates a landmark that the surgeon chose to help determine the AVM's location. The green and blue arrow indicate two veins that correspond to the veins seen in the AR view (right). *Centre:* Live image from the camera of the patient's dura. *Right:* Augmented reality view with camera image overlaid on volume rendered vessels, some edges are retained from the camera image. The white arrow indicates the green sphere/area of interest. The blue and green arrows correspond to the indicated veins in the left images of this figure.

abnormal connections occur within or between tough dural layers where rupture is unlikely, the bleeding risk arises due to the high pressure, extradural, cortical venous reflux component. Arteriovenous fistulas can be treated either by means of endovascular embolization of the arterial feeders and nidus, or by surgical means where the fistula nidus is isolated from its arterial feeders and veins draining to the brain.

Our AR system was brought into surgery in a 52 year old male with a type II Borden dural AV fistula (post embolization). The dural AV fistula was mainly supplied by the dorsal clival artery of the left internal carotid artery and recurrent lacrimal branch from the left ophthalmic artery which drains into the spinous branch from the left middle meningeal artery and drained by the left petrosal vein in the left CP angle cistern and eventually via a cortical vein into the right basal vein of Rosenthal.

In our third surgical case, there was a significant improvement in terms of the visualization of vessels. Edges of the vessels were visualized, giving a perception of relative depth. As we had both an arterial and venous phase DS CTA we could use colour-coding to differentiate between veins and arteries (see Fig 5). The colour-coding was changed from previous cases (red/purple) to colours that would help differentiate the augmented images from the surrounding anatomy and blood (i.e., purple, yellow-green, and orange). The surgeon commented on the improved contrast from the new colour paradigm saying it was easier to understand the augmented view.

During this case, we acquired several images prior to resection on top of the dura (Fig 5) and also during resection. However, in both sequences of camera images the vessels are not easily identifiable in the images. Looking at the augmented reality view, the surgeon commented on the fact that the system, similar to the commercial system was off by about 2mm in the sagittal plane after significant resection. This can be partially attributed to the fact that the

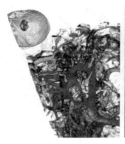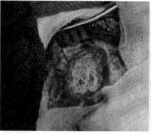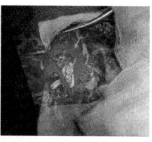

Fig. 5. *Left:* Cerebral vasculature of patient from an arterial phase (orange) and venous phase (purple) DS CTA and green-yellow for vessels around the fistula. The green arrow indicates the transverse sinus and pink indicates the fistula. *Centre:* A live image of the patient's dura after craniotomy during neurovascular surgery. *Right:* An AR view showing segmented vessels.

patient's preoperative images were from a much earlier date and the patient was not rescanned prior to surgery. The results of this case were limited by the fact that there was little space in the OR theatre and that the camera could not be brought close enough to the patient's anatomy because of safety (sterility) reasons. To improve further on our current progress we will need to acquire images closer to the anatomy where more detail can be seen.

6   Discussion and Conclusions

We have successfully brought our AR system into the OR and have had positive feedback about the use of augmented reality to aid in surgery, particularily in terms of localization of regions of interest in the vasculature and for planning of the craniotomy, the dural opening and the resection corridor. We are currently focusing on improving the system based on the comments from surgeons within the OR and discussions with the surgeons after each surgical case. In particular we are working to address the augmented reality visualization of the vessels and on improving the workflow by directly augmenting the microscope image.

We are currently working on more robust ways to filter the live-camera image and improve visualization of the vessels, particularly in terms of depth perception. Due to the fact that the camera is external and cannot be used while the neurosurgical microscope is in use we have only images before the opening of the dura or after significant amounts of resection, i.e. close to the end of surgery. We found that our AR visualization on top of the dura allowed surgeons to understand the topology of the vessels below the surface and helped them to plan a corridor of resection towards an area of interest. Localization can also be extremely important for particular tasks or under certain circumstances.

In terms of depth perception and understanding vessel topology, it is likely that a number of our visualization techniques may perform better when more of the cortex is visible as the images will be less contaminated by blood and vessels on the cortex can be delineated better. At the same time, it is important

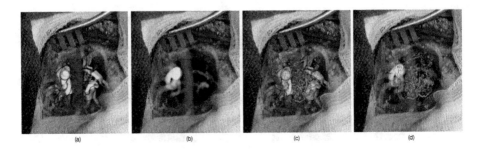

Fig. 6. Volume rendered vessels (purple vessels for venous phase, orange vessels for arterial phase and green/yellow vessels for the vessels around the fistual) from Case 3. (a) Vessels directly alpha blended with the camera image. The vessels seem to float above or on the surface of the patient. (b) Using the depth cue of fog to show distance. Vessels that exhibit less opacity/are more faded are further away from the surface of the brain. (c) Volume rendered vessels and retained edges from the camera image. The vessels now appear below the surface. (d) Rendered vessels using fog and retaining edges from the camera image. This type of visualization begins to give a sense of the relative depth of vessels within the brain.

to develop visualization techniques that are effective at different times within the surgery and not only when images are ideal.

In Fig. 6 we post-operatively explored a few visualization techniques. We find that edges help improve the perception that the virtual object is within the patient's brain, and that fog gives a better overall impression of depth, and in particular relative depth. Furthermore, it reduces the complexity of the scene by not showing vessels that are far away from the patient surface. For surgical tasks that require a better understanding of the topology and in particular the depth of vessels below the surface better visualization techniques are needed. In future work we will look at non-photorealistic rendering of vessels, decluttering, and using grids or rulers to show depth.

In terms of *visualization processing*, our experiences show that we are not able to quickly work on changing the visualization properties on the fly in the OR. This is due to the fact that the use of our system is minimized as it causes an interruption to workflow. One solution would be able to improve the *interface* to be able to change between visualization techniques with click of the button, rather than tune transfer functions, opacity, edges, on the fly. Another possibility is to use simpler visualization techniques, for certain surgical tasks. This is something we will explore in future work.

In terms of hardware and *display*, the next step of this work, will be to improve on our system by augmenting the microscope image directly, rather than having an external camera, which causes interruptions to the surgical workflow. Images from a neurosurgical microscope will enable augmentation of the view at any point during surgery.

The main contribution of this work is the description of our experiences in bringing in a research augmented reality neuronavigation system into the OR.

As with any software system, design and evaluation is cyclical. We have brought in our system into the OR three times, and each time we have improved on our previous experiences. By sharing our experiences and conclusions we aim to aid others in moving from use of an AR system in the laboratory to use in the OR.

Acknowledgments. This work was financed by the FQRNT, CIHR (MOP-97820), NSERC, and the Dejardins Group.

References

1. Birkfellner, W., Figl, M., Huber, K., Watzinger, F., Wanschitz, F., Hummel, J., Hanel, R., Greimel, W., Homolka, P., Ewers, R., Bergmann, H.: A head-mounted operating binocular for augmented reality visualization in medicine–design and initial evaluation. IEEE TMI 21(8), 991–997 (2002)
2. Cabrilo, I., Bijlenga, P., Schaller, K.: Augmented Reality in the Surgery of Cerebral Aneurysms: A Technical Report. Neurosurgery 10, 252–261 (2014)
3. Drouin, S., Kersten-Oertel, M., Chen, S.J.-S., Collins, D.L.: A Realistic Test and Development Environment for Mixed Reality in Neurosurgery. In: Linte, C.A., Moore, J.T., Chen, E.C.S., Holmes III, D.R. (eds.) AE-CAI 2011. LNCS, vol. 7264, pp. 13–23. Springer, Heidelberg (2012)
4. Edwards, P.J., King, A.P., Hawkes, D.J., Fleig, O., Maurer Jr., C.R., Hill, D.L., Fenlon, M.R., de Cunha, D.A., Gaston, R.P., Chandra, S., Mannss, J., Strong, A.J., Gleeson, M.J., Cox, T.C.: Stereo Augmented Reality in the Surgical Microscope. Stud. Health Technol. Inform. 62, 102–108 (1999)
5. Kersten-Oertel, M., Chen, S.J.S., Collins, D.L.: An Evaluation of Depth Enhancing Perceptual Cues for Vascular Volume Visualization in Neurosurgery. IEEE TVCG 20(3), 391–403 (2014)
6. Kersten-Oertel, M., Jannin, P., Collins, D.L.: The state of the art of visualization in mixed reality image guided surgery. CMIG 37(2), 98–112 (2013)
7. Kersten-Oertel, M., Jannin, P., Collins, D.L.: DVV: A Taxonomy for Mixed Reality Visualization in Image Guided Surgery. IEEE TVCG 18(2), 332–352 (2012)
8. Kersten-Oertel, M., Drouin, S., Chen, S.J.S., Collins, D.L.: Augmented Reality Visualization for Guidance in Neurovascular Surgery. Stud. Health Technol. Inform. 173, 225–229 (2012)
9. Paul, P., Fleig, O., Jannin, P.: Augmented Virtuality Based on Stereoscopic Reconstruction in Multimodal Image-Guided Neurosurgery: Methods and Performance Evaluation. IEEE TMI 24(11), 1500–1511 (2005)

A New Cost-Effective Approach to Pedicular Screw Placement

Jonas Walti[1], Gregory F. Jost[2], and Philippe C. Cattin[1]

[1] MIAC, Dep. Biomedical Engineering, University of Basel, Switzerland
[2] Department of Neurosurgery, University Hospital of Basel, Switzerland

Abstract. The placement of pedicle screws in open spine surgery is difficult. Warranting the correct trajectory is crucial because a wrongly placed screw will lead to a bad fit or will harm the patient's neurovascular structure. Current state of the art techniques are based on the surgeon's experience and multiple fluoroscopic images or an expensive and complex intraoperative navigation system.

This paper describes a novel method which is intended to support the surgeon during the insertion of pedicle screws in a simple yet cost-effective and reliable way. The approach uses inertial measurement sensors to track the pose of the surgical instruments and a software application for visualization and guiding. In a pre-clinical cadaver study a performance of 74 out of 80 clinically correctly placed screws has been reached without the use of any fluoroscopic images.

Keywords: Inertial Navigation System, Spinal Instrumentation.

1   Introduction

Spinal instrumentation describes a surgical procedure to implant metallic or non-metallic devices into the spine. Typically, these implants consist of plates, rods and screws to connect parts of the spine. The goal of such a surgery is usually to restore stability or to correct deformations (like scoliosis) of the spine.

Warranting the correct trajectory to implant a screw without harming neurovascular structures depends on obtaining a pathway with the correct starting point and tilt in the sagittal and axial plane. In open spine surgery, the starting point is defined by exposed anatomic landmarks, but the level within the spine and sagittal tilt of the vertebral body with respect to the surgical instruments and their advancement into the bone are usually controlled with intraoperative lateral fluoroscopy. The axial tilt is commonly chosen by feel and experience after looking at the preoperative imaging data. Hence, the procedure is associated with considerable subjective control. Contemporary image guidance tracks the position of surgical tools in relation to the anatomy and renders a real-time visualization in three planes on the screen of a workstation. These devices are excellent tools which may improve accuracy of spinal instrumentation [1,5] and reduce radiation exposure to the OR staff [6] and possibly the patient. However,

C.A. Linte et al. (Eds.): AE-CAI 2014, LNCS 8678, pp. 90–97, 2014.
© Springer International Publishing Switzerland 2014

their high cost (500000 - 750000 USD) precludes availability to most surgeons [2,7]. For this reason we have started to investigate alternative means of intra-operative navigation based on measuring tilt angles. This concept builds on the fact that full navigation support is not required for pedicular screw placement, as the starting point for the screw can easily be found by respecting anatomic landmarks. Similar to a simplified variant of the idea [3], we developed a navigation device based on an *inertial measurement unit (IMU)* that is attached to the surgical tools like the pedicle finder or the screwdriver. The mounted sensor device communicates wirelessly with a computer on which the orientation of the tool can be visualized and compared to the planned angles. This information allows real-time guidance to support the surgeon during screw placement.

2   Method

The proposed approach bases on the observation that for pedicular screw placement only the lateral and axial tilt angle need to be navigated. This results in a simple surgical procedure as described below in Figure 1.

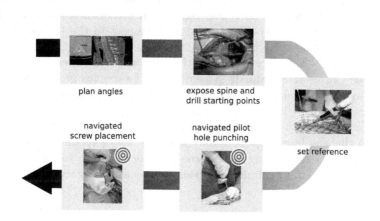

Fig. 1. Different steps for IMU-based navigated screw placement

2.1   Surgical Procedure

Angle Planning. As a first step, the surgeon has to define the insertion angles for the screws into the pedicle. Therefore, he plans for every single screw the exact angles on the transversal (axial angle) and sagittal plane (sagittal angle) from a preoperative 3D CT dataset and the help of an image viewer software like the *OsiriX* suite. The surgeon measures the angles for the screw with respect to a well defined and distinctive anatomical landmark edge. Because of its exposed structure, this is usually the *spinous process*, which is well visible in the CT image and during open spine surgery (see Fig. 2 and 3).

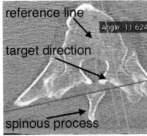
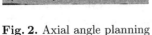
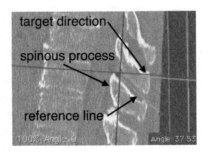

Fig. 2. Axial angle planning   **Fig. 3.** Sagittal angle planning

Intraoperative Entry Point Priming. Equivalent to all pedicular screw placement approaches, the entry point of the screw has to be decorticated first. This is done by removing the cortical bone with for example a drill.

Referencing of the Vertebral Body. To navigate the surgical tools, the reference coordinate system has to be defined first. This is done by simply aligning the navigated tool along the reference edge, which was defined during planning. As the target angles are usually planned with respect to the spinous process, see Fig. 4, the tool needs to be aligned parallel to this well defined anatomical landmark and recorded as reference by the software. This operation defines a right-handed Cartesian coordinate system where the spinous process defines the y-base-vector. The xy-plane lies completely in the body's sagittal plane. Therefore, the z-axis points in lateral direction. The sagittal angle is now defined between the y-axis of the reference coordinate system and the tool vector, projected onto the xy-plane. For the axial angle, the tool's vector is projected on the yz-plane. This referencing step is the equivalent to the tedious and often time consuming natural landmark selection in classical navigation solutions.

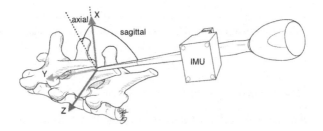

Fig. 4. This sketch shows the IMU-equipped pedicle finder aligned with the vertrebra's spinous process. This is the reference position. Note the two visualized angles.

Screw Placement. Once the vertebra is referenced, the pedicle finder is applied to drill a pilot hole. The tool is equipped with the mentioned IMU-based measuring device. This makes it possible to calculate and visualize the surgical tool's current tilt angles. The software guides the surgeon in real-time to the correct angulation for the pedicle finder with respect to the planned target angles. The same referencing and guiding process can also be used for a screwdriver equipped with the sensory device, which allows to insert the pedicle screws fully navigated.

2.2 Hardware

After some tests with different IMU-based products, the *MTw* sensor by *Xsens*[1] was chosen as measuring device. To calculate the orientation data, it uses a combination of highly sensitive MEMS-components, namely an accelerometer, a gyrosensor and a magnetometer per axis. An integrated CPU fuses the raw data of these sensors with an update rate of 1800 Hz to a final 3D-orientation output. The data is transmitted with an update rate of up to 120 Hz to a 2.4 GHz receiver-dongle, connected to a computer. According to the manufacturer the static accuracy of the final orientation-output is 0.5° for the pan and the tilt axes and 1° for the heading axis. The sensor costs around 2500 USD.

2.3 Sensor to Tool Calibration

The calibration step is needed to align the mounted sensors' coordinate system with the one of the surgical tool. If this is not the case, rotations around the tool's main axis would lead to wrong results. Because of the fact that all the measurements rely on relative rotations only and completely neglect any translations, a straightforward calibration routine was developed. When the tool is rotated mechanically guided around its main axis by 360°, every 120° the tool's main axis vector is collected (v_1, v_2 and v_3). With a perfectly aligned sensor, these vectors would all point into the same direction. But if the mounted sensor's internal coordinate system is slightly tilted as compared to the one of surgical tool, these vectors form a cone around the desired axis. With these three vectors, the transformation matrix $_TT^{TC}$ between the tool's coordinate system and the mounted sensor's coordinate system can be found (see Eq. 1). With such an exact calibration, the navigated surgical tool can be rotated around its main axis without influencing the calculated tilt angles during the navigation process. This calibration routine has to be executed only when the position of the sensor relative to the surgical tool has changed and takes about one minute.

$$
\begin{aligned}
C_x &= V_{x1} \times V_{x2} \quad \text{with} \quad V_{x1} = v_2' - v_1' \quad \text{and} \quad V_{x2} = v_3' - v_1' \\
C_y &= V_{y1} \times V_{y2} \quad \text{with} \quad V_{y1} = v_2 - v_1 \quad \text{and} \quad V_{y2} = v_3 - v_1 \\
C_z &= C_x \times C_y
\end{aligned}
$$

$$
_TT^{TC} = \begin{bmatrix} C_{x1} & C_{y1} & C_{z1} & 0 \\ C_{x2} & C_{y2} & C_{z2} & 0 \\ C_{x3} & C_{y3} & C_{z3} & 0 \\ 0 & 0 & 0 & 1 \end{bmatrix}
\tag{1}
$$

[1] www.xsens.com

The collected vectors v_1, v_2 and v_3 are rotated by 90° around the z-axis to get v_1', v_2', v_3'. With these additional vectors, the two vectors V_{x1}, V_{x2} which lie on a plane perpendicular to the x-axis can be found. The same is done for the y-axis (V_{y1}, V_{y2}). The transformation matrix' components C_x and C_y are calculated with the cross product of V_{x1} and V_{x2} respectively V_{y1} and V_{y2}. The matrix' missing C_z components are calculated with the cross product of the two already found vectors.

2.4   Angle Calculation

With the IMU-sensor's data, we are able to calculate the surgical tool's sagittal ($\alpha_{current}$) and axial ($\beta_{current}$) tilt angles with respect to the defined reference orientation. To avoid gimbal lock problems, the IMU-sensor's output data is used in the quaternion format. The provided quaternion is transferred into the 4 by 4 transformation matrix $_WT^T$. This matrix represents the tool's current orientation in arbitrary world coordinates, depending on the IMU-sensor's internal coordinate system. Thus, this matrix has to be transformed into the reference coordinate system $_WT^R$, defined by the surgeon during the referencing procedure. Furthermore, if there exists a calibration matrix $_TT^{TC}$ for the currently tracked surgical tool, the sensor's native coordinates have to be transferred into the tool's calibrated coordinate system first. See Eq. 2 for the final *raw sensor coordinates* to *calibrated tool coordinates* in the surgeon-defined *reference coordinate system* transformation $_RT^{TC}$.

$$_RT^{TC} = (_WT^R)^{-1} \cdot {_WT^T} \cdot {_TT^{TC}} \tag{2}$$

After these transformations have been applied, the resulting matrix $_RT^{TC}$ can be used to calculate the current orientation T of the tool's main axis T_{base} with respect to the defined reference coordinate system (Eq. 3). The current axial and sagittal angles are then calculated by projecting the tool vector T onto the xy-plane of the reference coordinate system for the sagittal angle (this leads to T_{noZ}) and onto the yz-plane for the axial angle (T_{noX}). For each of these two projected vectors, the dot product is used to calculate the final angles between the reference coordinate system's y-axis (Y_{base}) and the two projected vectors (Eq. 4 and 5).

$$T = T_{base} \cdot {_RT^{TC}} \tag{3}$$

$$\alpha_{current} = \arccos\left(\frac{Y_{base} \cdot T_{noZ}}{||Y_{base}|| \cdot ||T_{noZ}||}\right) \quad \text{with} \quad T_{noZ} = T \cdot \begin{bmatrix} 1 \\ 1 \\ 0 \end{bmatrix} \tag{4}$$

$$\beta_{current} = \arccos\left(\frac{Y_{base} \cdot T_{noX}}{||Y_{base}|| \cdot ||T_{noX}||}\right) \quad \text{with} \quad T_{noX} = T \cdot \begin{bmatrix} 0 \\ 1 \\ 1 \end{bmatrix} \tag{5}$$

3   Experiments and Results

3.1   Drift Measurements

To quantitatively evaluate the IMU sensor's accuracy over time, a comparative experiment with an optical tracking system (Axios[2]) was made as these systems are known to be very precise with a high repeatability. As the inertial measurement unit's errors accumulate over time, it was very important to know how accurate the measured values are after a certain period. To gather the values for these tests, an optical marker was rigidly attached to an IMU-sensor mounted on a surgical tool. The software's output angles at different orientations and different times were compared. See Table 1 for the results. The comparison of the measured angles shows that the gathered values are stable in the range of two degrees over a time period of at least 4.5 min for both angles. This duration is sufficient as the surgeon uses the tool for roughly one minute after the referencing step.

Table 1. This table shows the measured values at different orientations and times

| Time | Sagittal | | | Axial | | |
| | Optical | IMU | Error | Optical | IMU | Error |
[s]	[°]	[°]	[°]	[°]	[°]	[°]
30	24.8	25.9	1.1	24.3	23.7	0.6
60	21.9	21.4	0.5	27.3	29.3	2
90	22	21.4	0.6	27.1	26.5	0.6
120	34.6	34.7	0.1	9.7	9.9	0.2
150	31.2	31.2	0	10.2	9.3	0.9
180	10.1	9.2	0.9	18.7	19.5	0.8
210	30.7	30.1	0.6	16.2	16.1	0.1
240	17.1	15.5	1.6	22.2	22.2	0
270	17.2	15.6	1.6	22.4	22.5	0.1

3.2   Cadaver Experiments

To check the method's accuracy and usability, four trials with human cadavers were made. An experienced neurosurgeon led these experiments and set up a realistic approach and environment to execute the previously described steps of the method. The spine was exposed and the screw's entry points decorticated for the thoracic (T1 to T12) and the lumbosacral (L1 to S1) vertebrae. For each vertebra, one screw was inserted freehand and one using the proposed technique. To avoid any bias, after every six vertebrae the method's sides were switched from freehand to guided. For both approaches, no intraoperative fluoroscopic images were acquired. At the end of every experiment, two S2-ilium screws have

---

[2] www.axios3d.com

been placed additionally. Because it is virtually impossible to place these screws freehand without fluoroscopic images, they were applied with the IMU-navigated method on both sides.

When comparing the preoperatively planned angle with the post-operative measured angle a mean error of 2.7° for the axial and 3.5° for the sagittal angle has been observed for the 80 screws applied with the proposed IMU-based technique. This is more accurate than the neurosurgeon's freehand approach with a mean error of 4.1° (axial) and 6° (sagittal) for 72 screws, see Table 2. A one sided t-test shows p-values of 0.00287 (axial) and 0.00088 (sagittal) confirming that the freehand method performs worse for both angles than the newly developed navigated approach.

Besides the quantitative evaluation, the final positions of the screws were also compared in terms of clinical correctness. A screw was classified as clinically correct if it lies completely in the pedicle without any perforation. With the navigated method 74 out of 80 (93%) screws were placed clinically correct whereas 64 of 72 (89%) were applied clinically correct with the freehand method. Other clinical studies report success rates between 68% and 90% for the standard freehand approach supported by additional fluoroscopic images [5].

Table 2. The comparison of the trial results

| Cadaver [Number] | IMU-navigated | | | Freehand | | |
	Error Axial [°]	Sagittal [°]	Clinically Correct [#Screws]	Error Axial [°]	Sagittal [°]	Clinically Correct [#Screws]
I	2.5	3.2	19/20 (95%)	2.9	5.1	16/18 (89%)
II	3.4	4	16/20 (80%)	3.4	5.3	15/18 (83)%
III	2.5	3.7	19/20 (95%)	4.9	9.9	16/18 (89%)
IV	2.4	3.1	20/20 (100%)	5.2	3.7	17/18 (94%)
Overall	**2.7**	**3.5**	**74/80 (93%)**	**4.1**	**6.0**	**64/72 (89%)**

4   Discussion and Conclusion

The sensor's accuracy and drift tests showed errors in the range of zero to two degrees. On the other hand, the errors of the applied screws' final positions were slightly higher. One reason for this may be the manually executed process for planning and reviewing the screws' directions. It is difficult to define the target angles and read out the final angles with the exact same reference. Another source of possible inaccuracies is the referencing step. Depending on the spine's anatomy it is not always easy to align the tool to the same reference as the one defined during the planning step. Errors of up to three degrees have to be expected there. But because of the spine's anatomy, errors in these ranges do still lead to clinically correctly placed screws, which is the most important measure in real surgery. To apply a screw a mean duration of 2.5 minutes was reached. This underlines the method's excellent performance in effectiveness and simplicity. It shows that the implemented software guidance suits the surgeon's demands in the field and that the whole method is reasonable and straightforward. A furthermore advantage of the newly proposed method is that no line-of-sight restrictions are given and that there is no need to attach bulky markers onto the surgical tools and the spine itself. As each vertebra is referenced individually the approach can also nicely handle deformed vertebrae or scoliotic patients. It overcomes most of the currently used image guided methods' problems also mentioned in a recent publication by Amir Manbachi et al. [4].

Additionally, the proposed approach proved to be efficient and accurate for placing the S2-ilium screw connecting the sacrum with the pelvis bone. This 10 cm long screw is very demanding to place with the freehand method and does generally require the use of multiple fluoroscopic images.

In the future we plan to reduce the cost of the device further, simplify the planning procedure and possibly also perform a pilot clinical study.

References

1. Chiang, C.-Y.F., Tsai, T.-T., Chen, L.-H., Lai, P.-L., Fu, T.-S., Niu, C.-C., Chen, W.-J.: Computed tomography-based navigation-assisted pedicle screw insertion for thoracic and lumbar spine fractures. Chang Gung Med. J. 35(4), 332-8 (2012)
2. Costa, F., Cardia, A., Ortolina, A., Fabio, G., Zerbi, A., Fornari, M.: Spinal navigation: standard preoperative versus intraoperative computed tomography data set acquisition for computer-guidance system: radiological and clinical study in 100 consecutive patients. Spine 36(24), 2094–2098 (2011)
3. Jost, G.F., Bisson, E.F., Schmidt, M.H.: ipod touch®-assisted instrumentation of the spine: A technical report. Neurosurgery (2013)
4. Manbachi, A., Cobbold, R.S., Ginsberg, H.J.: Guided pedicle screw insertion: techniques and training. The Spine Journal 14(1), 165–179 (2014)
5. Mason, A., Paulsen, R., Babuska, J.M., Rajpal, S., Burneikiene, S., Nelson, E.L., Villavicencio, A.T.: The accuracy of pedicle screw placement using intraoperative image guidance systems: A systematic review. Journal of Neurosurgery: Spine, 1–8 (2013)
6. Smith, H.E., Welsch, M.D., Sasso, R.C., Vaccaro, A.R.: Comparison of radiation exposure in lumbar pedicle screw placement with fluoroscopy vs computer-assisted image guidance with intraoperative three-dimensional imaging. J. Spinal Cord Med. 31, 532–537 (2008)
7. Watkins IV, R.G., Gupta, A., Watkins III, R.G.: Cost-effectiveness of image-guided spine surgery. The Open Orthopaedics Journal 4, 228 (2010)

A Simple and Accurate Camera-Sensor Calibration for Surgical Endoscopes and Microscopes

Seongpung Lee[1], Hyunki Lee[2], Hyunseok Choi[1], and Jaesung Hong[1]

[1] Daegu Gyeongbuk Institute of Science and Technology, Robotics Engineering, Daegu, Korea
[2] Koh Young Technology, Medical Robot Unit, Seoul, Korea
jhong@dgist.ac.kr

Abstract. Nowadays, augmented reality (AR) has become a key technology for surgical navigation. It is necessary to perform camera-sensor calibration to build AR between a camera and a sensor that tracks the camera. In order to perform camera-sensor calibration, it has been common method to move the camera in such a way as to solve an $AX = XB$ type formula. However, in clinical environments, Endoscopes and microscopes are commonly used, and moving those cameras is very difficult due to their large weight and size when camera-sensor calibration is performed. Therefore, we propose a method to solve the camera-sensor matrix by expanding the $AX = XB$ equation to the $AX = BYC$ equation. Instead of moving the camera, we move the calibration pattern in the proposed method. Through the experiments, we compared the $AX = BYC$ solution with the $AX = XB$ solution in terms of the accuracy. As a result, we found the proposed method is more convenient and accurate than the conventional method.

Keywords: Camera Calibration, Hand-Eye Calibration, Surgical Endoscopes, Surgical Microscopes.

1   Introduction

Conventional surgical navigation systems provide only information about where the surgical tool is in the patient with multi-planar display and graphic objects in virtual space. However, in augmented-reality-based surgical navigation, the shape of invisible organs are overlapped to the endoscopic or microscopic images, allowing the surgeon to intuitively recognize the target organ position and reduce the incision area [1]. The optical tracker and the camera are commonly used for AR-based surgery, as shown in Fig. 1. In order to build an AR-based surgical navigation system, it is necessary to perform two steps of calibration, which are camera-sensor calibration and camera calibration. Camera calibration is the process to obtain intrinsic parameters, which consist of focal length, principal point, etc., and is used for setting the properties of a virtual camera. Zhang's camera calibration method has been commonly used to perform camera calibration because it provides high accuracy and is easy to use [2]. Camera-sensor calibration is identical in theory to hand-eye calibration in robotics. Hand-eye calibration is known as the $AX = XB$ problem, and the solution is a

C.A. Linte et al. (Eds.): AE-CAI 2014, LNCS 8678, pp. 98–107, 2014.
© Springer International Publishing Switzerland 2014

transformation matrix from the end-effector to the camera lens [3,4,5,6]. By using the result of hand-eye calibration, i.e. camera-sensor calibration the virtual camera can be located in same position as the real one. This camera-sensor calibration affects the overall accuracy of AR [7]. In this study, we propose a simple and accurate method using AX=BYC relationship instead of AX=XB to find a camera-sensor matrix.

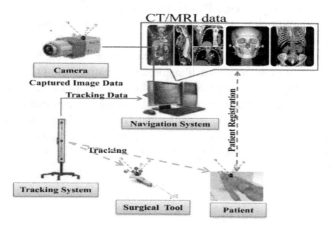

Fig. 1. Schematic of AR-based surgical navigation system. In order to build an AR system, an optical tracker and camera are used in medical applications.

In Chapter 2, we will briefly explain two conventional approaches to solve the AX = BYC problem that were firstly introduced by Aiguo Li [8]. In addition, we will present two methods to perform hand-eye calibration. One is to move the camera, as with the conventional method. The other is to move the calibration pattern, as we propose. In Chapter 3, we compare results of each method by using re-projection error, and we draw conclusions in Chapter 4. We will use the well-known terminology, hand-eye calibration instead of the camera-sensor calibration throughout this article.

2   Methods

2.1   Definition of the AX = BYC Problem

In the conventional $AX = XB$ problem, A and B are obtained by moving the camera pose several times, where A is obtained from two transformations between the robot base and the end-effector of a robot arm, B is obtained from two transformations between the camera lens and the calibration pattern, and X is defined for the relationship of the end-effector of the robot arm to the camera lens, as shown in Fig. 2(a).

In AR-based surgical navigation, the optical tracker (OT) and the passive marker affixed to the camera (CM) can be regarded as the robot base and the end-effector, respectively. Therefore, in order to perform hand-eye calibration, the surgeon have to move the camera manually unless there is any automatic system to perform hand-eye calibration. However, it is very difficult for the surgeon to move the camera since endoscopes and microscopes are often heavy and large. If the $AX = XB$ problem is expanded to the $AX = BYC$ problem by attaching an additional passive marker on the calibration pattern (PM), as shown in Fig. 2 (b), it is easier than the aforementioned case to perform hand-eye calibration since it is possible to move the calibration pattern instead of the heavy camera. This problem is very similar to the $AX = ZB$ and $AX = YB$ problems introduced by [8,9,10,11]; however, they do not move the calibration pattern to solve the problem.

In the $AX = BYC$ problem, the meaning of each notation is slightly different from that of the $AX = XB$ problem. A is a transformation matrix from OT to CM, B is the one from OT to PM, C is the one from the calibration pattern to the camera lens, Y is the one from PM to the calibration pattern, and X is the same as that of the $AX = XB$ problem, i.e. the transform matrix from the end-effector of the robot arm to the camera lens. As shown in Fig. 2 (b), the equation is more intuitive than $AX = XB$ since the $AX = BYC$ problem is established from one pose while the $AX = XB$ problem is established from two poses.

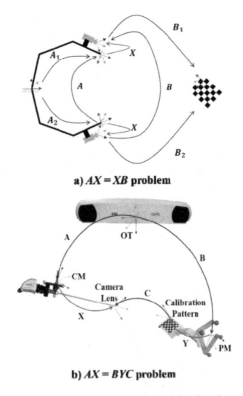

a) $AX = XB$ problem

b) $AX = BYC$ problem

Fig. 2. Conventional method and proposed method for solving hand-eye calibration. The upper figure shows the conventional method in robotics applications. In such applications, the A and B matrices can be obtained from two poses. However, in the lower figure, which describes the proposed method, A, B, and C matrices can be obtained from only one pose.

2.2   Two Previous Approaches to Solve the AX = BYC Problem

In the $AX = XB$ problem, dual quaternion and Kronecker product approaches have been developed to solve the rotation and translation parts simultaneously [4,12]. In the $AX = BYC$ problem, those two approaches are modified to solve X and Y simultaneously. The other way to solve that problem is to solve X and Y separately. However, if X and Y are solved separately, the error of Y affects the accuracy of X when X is calculated. In the following two subsections, we briefly explain two conventional approaches to solve the $AX = BYC$ problem that can be simply derived from the original equation.

Dual Quaternion Approach. Dual Quaternion, $\hat{q}$ defined as Eq. (1).

$$\hat{q} = q + \varepsilon\, q', \tag{1}$$

where q is a unit quaternion defined as Eq. (2), q' is a quaternion defined as Eq. (3), and ε is a dual unit in which $\varepsilon^2 = 0$.

$$q = \sin\left(\frac{\theta}{2}\right) l + \cos\left(\frac{\theta}{2}\right), \tag{2}$$

where θ is the rotation angle about the rotation axis, and l is a unit vector with same direction to the rotation axis.

$$q' = -\frac{q^T t}{2} + \frac{t q_0}{2} t \times \boldsymbol{q}, \tag{3}$$

where q_0 is a scalar of unit quaternion, $\boldsymbol{q}$ is a vector part of the unit quaternion, and t is translation. Therefore, if the transformation matrix is known, it can be converted from 4-by-4 matrix form to dual quaternion form. First, in order to derive an $AX = BYC$ equation by using the dual quaternion, multiply each side by the inverse of B. Then, let $B^{-1}A$ define D. After that, let $\hat{q}_D, \hat{q}_C, \hat{q}_X$, and $\hat{q}_Y$ be dual-quaternion for D, C, X, and Y, respectively. Then Eq. (4) will be obtained.

$$\hat{q}_D \hat{q}_X = \hat{q}_Y \hat{q}_C \tag{4}$$

By using dual quaternion definition Eq. (1), Eq. (4) can be separately rewritten as Eq. (5) and Eq. (6).

$$dx = yc \tag{5}$$

$$d'x + dx' = yc' + y'c \tag{6}$$

Eq. (5) and Eq. (6) can be expressed in matrix form. Therefore, Eq. (5) and Eq. (6) can be rewritten as Eq. (7) and Eq. (8).

$$\tilde{d}x - \check{c}y = 0 \tag{7}$$

$$\tilde{d}'x + \tilde{d}x' - \tilde{c}'y - \check{c}y' = 0 \tag{8}$$

Therefore,

$$\begin{bmatrix} \tilde{d} & 0_{4\times4} & \tilde{c} & 0_{4\times4} \\ \tilde{d}' & \tilde{d} & -\tilde{c}' & -\tilde{c} \end{bmatrix} \begin{bmatrix} x \\ x' \\ y \\ y' \end{bmatrix} = 0 \tag{9}$$

8×16 matrix in Eq. (9) is generally defined as the S_i matrix, where i is the index for poses. At least two poses are needed for solving Eq. (9). When the number of poses is larger than two, Eq. (9) can be rewritten as Eq. (10).

$$[S_1, \quad S_2, \quad \cdots, \quad S_n]^T \begin{bmatrix} x \\ x' \\ y \\ y' \end{bmatrix} = 0 \tag{10}$$

We define $T = [S_1, \quad S_2, \quad \cdots, \quad S_n]^T$. By decomposing T with a singular value decomposition method (SVD), X and Y can be obtained.

Kronecker Product Approach. Kronecker product is defined as Eq. (11).

$$A \otimes B = [a_{ij}B] = \begin{bmatrix} a_{11}B & \cdots & a_{1n}B \\ \vdots & \ddots & \vdots \\ a_{m1}B & \cdots & a_{mn}B \end{bmatrix} \tag{11}$$

In addition to that definition, a stack operator is used in this solution. A stack operator is defined as Eq. (12).

$$\text{Vec}(A_{n\times m}) = [a_{11}, a_{12}, \cdots, a_{1n}, \cdots, a_{mn}]^T \tag{12}$$

Let $AX = BYC$ be $DX = YC$, where $D = B^{-1}A$. $DX = YC$ can be separated to a rotation part and translation part as Eq. (13) and Eq. (14).

$$R_D R_X - R_Y R_C = 0 \tag{13}$$

$$R_D t_X - R_Y t_C - t_Y = t_D \tag{14}$$

By using the definitions of Eq. (11) and Eq. (12), Eq. (13) and Eq. (14) can be rewritten as Eq. (15) and (16).

$$[R_D \otimes I_{3\times3}][\text{Vec}(R_X)] - [I_{3\times3} \otimes R_C^T][\text{Vec}(R_Y)] = 0 \tag{15}$$

$$R_D t_X - [I_{3\times3} \otimes t_B^T][\text{Vec}(R_Y)] - t_Y = t_D \tag{16}$$

Therefore,

$$\begin{bmatrix} R_D \otimes I_{3\times3} & -I_{3\times3} \otimes R_C^T & 0_{9\times3} & 0_{9\times3} \\ 0_{3\times9} & -I_{3\times3} \otimes t_B^T & R_D & -I_{3\times3} \end{bmatrix} \begin{bmatrix} \text{Vec}(R_X) \\ \text{Vec}(R_Y) \\ t_X \\ t_Y \end{bmatrix} = \begin{bmatrix} 0_{9\times1} \\ t_D \end{bmatrix}. \tag{17}$$

The form of Eq. (17) has $Qv = p$. Q has dimensions of 12×24, v has dimensions of 24×1, and p has dimensions of 12×1. Q and p are the notations for one pose. If the number of poses is larger than 2, Eq. (17) can be rewritten as Eq. (18).

$$[Q_1, \quad Q_2, \quad \cdots, \quad Q_n]^T [v] = [p_1, \quad p_2, \quad \cdots, \quad p_n]^T \qquad (18)$$

We define $M = [Q_1, \quad Q_2, \quad \cdots, \quad Q_n]^T$ and $N = [p_1, \quad p_2, \quad \cdots, \quad p_n]^T$. By using the M and N matrices, Eq. (18) can be solved by pseudo inverse as Eq. (19).

$$v = (M^T M)^{-1} M^T N \qquad (19)$$

The rotation part of v has the noise. Therefore, a normalization step is needed for obtaining an orthogonal matrix. In order to normalize the rotation matrix, Rodrigues and SVD can be used.

2.3   Conventional and Proposed Method to Perform Hand-Eye Calibration

In order to solve the $AX = XB$ problem, as shown in Fig. 3(a), the camera is moved while the calibration pattern is not moved. However, if an additional position sensor marker is affixed to the calibration pattern, the $AX = XB$ problem can be expanded to the $AX = BYC$ problem, as shown in Fig. 3(b). In this case, it is possible to move the calibration pattern to perform the hand-eye calibration.

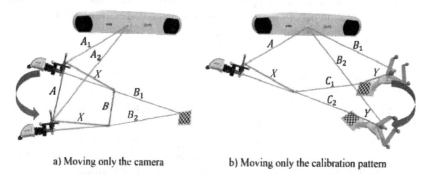

a) Moving only the camera   b) Moving only the calibration pattern

Fig. 3. Conventional method and proposed method to obtain the information relative to poses. The left figure shows the conventional method, and the right figure shows the proposed method.

2.4   Experiments

In this paper, experiments were performed to compare the proposed method with the conventional method. Experiments were conducted with an optical tracker system (Polaris Spectra, NDI, Canada) to track the position and the orientation of the passive marker, an endoscopic system (1188HD, STRYKER, USA) to capture the calibration pattern image, and the calibration pattern with dimensions of 7×6 which has 8.5×8.5 mm in each square. In case of the conventional method, the number of experiments was 20, and in each experiment, the pose information of the camera was acquired while it was moved to 30 locations with different orientation and position. Experiment setting for the proposed method was same as that of the conventional method except that the calibration pattern was moved instead of the camera. After performing hand-eye calibration by using the acquired data, in order to compare each method in terms of the accuracy, 100 images and poses obtained from moving both the camera and the calibration pattern and Eq. (20) was used. Eq. (20) represents the average re-projection error, ϵ.

$$\epsilon = \frac{1}{mn}\sum_{i=1}^{m}\sum_{j=1}^{n}\|p_i - p'_j\| \text{ (pixels)},$$ (20)

where m is the number of images we used in each experiment, n is the number of corner points of the calibration pattern, and p and p' are the corner points of the calibration pattern obtained from image processing by using m-th picture and the re-projection points obtained from Eq. (21), respectively.

$$\begin{bmatrix} p' \\ 1 \end{bmatrix} = \begin{bmatrix} f_x & 0 & c_x \\ 0 & f_y & c_y \\ 0 & 0 & 1 \end{bmatrix} [I_{3\times3}|0_{3\times1}][X^{-1} \quad A^{-1} \quad B \quad Y]\begin{bmatrix} P \\ 1 \end{bmatrix},$$ (21)

where p' is a 2D point in image coordinate, f_x, f_y are focal length, c_x, c_y are principal points, and P is a 3D corner point of the calibration pattern.

In addition, the ranges of motion of the camera and the calibration pattern were investigated to analyze the effect of the motions on the accuracy. The translation vectors were extracted from the acquired camera poses for the conventional method and the acquired poses of the calibration pattern for the proposed method, respectively. With the translation vectors, we plotted the motion range on the 3D graph (Figs. 6 and 7).

3   Experimental Results

Figs. 4 and 5 show the experimental results. In Figs. 4 and 5, MP and MC represent moving the calibration pattern and moving the camera respectively. The average and standard deviation were used to illustrate experimental results. As shown in Figs. 4 and 5, the accuracy of the proposed method was increased by approximately 33 pixels with Kronecker product approach, and 13 pixels with dual quaternion approach.

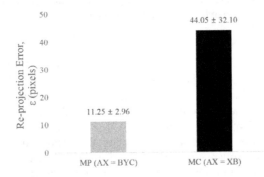

Fig. 4. Re-projection error of each method when using Kronecker product approach

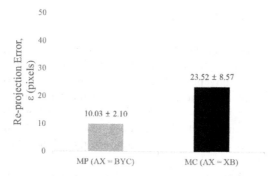

Fig. 5. Re-projection error of each method when using the dual quaternion approach

Fig. 6 shows the positions of the camera over 20 experiments in the conventional method. In the conventional method, the motion of the camera ranged from -800 mm to -1400 mm along z axis. Fig. 7 shows the position of the calibration pattern over 20 experiments in the proposed method. In the proposed method, the motion of the calibration pattern ranged from -1050 mm to -1150 mm along z axis. The range of the motion in the proposed method was smaller than that in the conventional one.

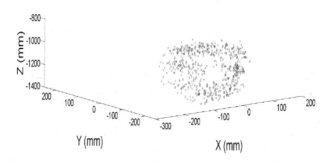

Fig. 6. Motion of the camera in the conventional method

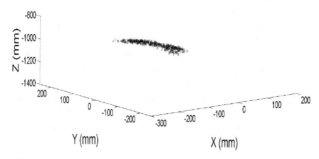

Fig. 7. Motion of the calibration pattern in the proposed method

4   Discussions and Conclusions

The aim of this study is to make hand-eye calibration easy and to improve the accuracy of hand-eye calibration by reducing the influence of optical tracker error. The proposed method is more convenient, because one can readily move the calibration pattern thanks to its light weight and small size without moving the heavy camera such as endoscopes or microscopes for the hand-eye calibration. Although the experiments were performed with the endoscope, the proposed method is also applicable to hand-eye calibration of microscopes since the mathematical model used in microscopes is same as that in endoscopes.

When hand-eye calibration was performed by using proposed method, the reprojection error was smaller than that of conventional method since it is possible to perform hand-eye calibration in a narrow workspace as shown in Fig. 7. A small range of movement of the pattern leads to increasing accuracy of hand-eye calibration since spatial error is increased when the distance between the passive marker and optical tracker is increased [13,14].

Acknowledgements. This work was supported by the Health and Medical R&D Program of the Ministry of Health and Welfare of Korea (HI13C1634) and by the Industrial Source Technology Development Program of the Ministry of Trade, Industry and Energy of Korea (10040097).

References

1. King, A.P., Edwards, P.J., Maurer, C.R., de Cunha, D.A., Gaston, R.P., Clarkson, M., Hill, D.L.G., Hawkes, D.J., Fenlon, M.R., Strong, A.J., Cox, T.C.S., Gleeson, M.J.: Stereo Augmented Reality in the surgical Microscope. Presence: Teleoperators and Virtual Environments 9(4), 360–368 (2000)
2. Zhang, Z.: A Flexible New Technique for Camera Calibration. IEEE Transactions on Pattern Analysis and Machine Intelligence 22(11), 1330–1334 (2000)
3. Tsai, R., Lenz, R.: A new technique for fully autonomous and efficient 3D robotics hand/eye calibration. IEEE Transactions on Robotics and Automation 5(3), 345–358 (1989)
4. Daniilidis, K.: Hand-Eye Calibration Using DualQuaternions. The International Journal of Robotics Research 18(3), 286–298 (1999)
5. Zhao, Z.: Hand-Eye Calibration Using ConvexOptimization. In: IEEE International Conference on Robotics and Automation, pp. 2947–2952 (2011)
6. Mao, J., Huang, X., Jiang, L.: A Flexible Solution toAX=XB for Robot Hand-Eye Calibration. In: Proceedings of the 10th WSEAS International Conference on Robotics, Control and Manufacturing Technology, pp. 118–122 (2010)
7. Bianchi, G., Harders, C.W.M., Cattin, P., Szekely, G.: Camera-marker alignment framework and comparison with hand-eye calibration for augmented reality applications. In: Proceedings of Fourth IEEE and ACM International Symposium on Mixed and Augmented Reality, pp. 188–189 (2005)

8. Aiguo, L., Lin, W., Defeng, W.: Simultaneous robot-world and hand-eye calibration using dual-quaternions and Kronecker product. International Journal of Physical Sciences 5(10), 1530–1536 (2010)
9. Zhuang, H., Roth, S., Sudhakar, R.: Simultaneous Robot/World and Tool/Flange Calibration by Solving Homogeneous Transformation Equations of the form AX=YB. IEEE Transactions on Robotics and Automation 10(4), 549–554 (1994)
10. Dornaika, F., Horaud, R.: Simultaneous robot-world and hand-eye calibration. IEEE Transactions onRobotics and Automation 14(4), 617–622 (1998)
11. Strobl, K.H., Hirzinger, G.: Optimal Hand-Eye Calibration. In: 2006 IEEE/RSJ International Conference on Intelligent Robots and Systems, pp. 4647–4653 (2006)
12. Andreff, N., Horaud, R., Espiau, B.: On-line Hand-Eye Calibration. In: Proceedings of Second International Conference on 3-D Digital Imaging and Modeling, pp. 430–436 (1999)
13. Wiles, A.D., Thompsona, D.G., Frantz, D.D.: Accuracy assessment and interpretation for optical tracking systems. In: Proc. of SPIE Medical Imaging, vol. 5367, pp. 421–432 (2004)
14. Koivukangas, T., Katisko, J., Koivukangas, J.: Technical accuracy of optical and the electromagnetic tracking systems. SpringerPlus 2(1), 1–7 (2013)

Augmented-Reality Environment for Locomotor Training in Children with Neurological Injuries*

Angelos Barmpoutis[1], Emily J. Fox[1], Ian Elsner[1], and Sheryl Flynn[2]

[1] University of Florida, Gainesville FL 32611, USA,
{angelos,ian}@digitalworlds.ufl.edu, ejfox@phhp.ufl.edu
[2] Blue Marble Game Co, Altadena CA 91001, USA
sheryl@bluemarblegameco.com

Abstract. In this paper a novel augmented-reality environment is presented for enhancing locomotor training. The main goal of this environment is to excite kids for walking and hence facilitate their locomotor therapy and at the same time provide the therapist with a quantitative framework for monitoring and evaluating the progress of the therapy. This paper focuses on the quantitative part of our framework, which uses a depth camera to capture the patient's body motion. More specifically, we present a model-free graph-based segmentation algorithm that detects the regions of the arms and legs in the depth frames. Then, we analyze their motion patterns in real-time by extracting various features such as the pace, length of stride, symmetry of walking pattern, and arm-leg synchronization. Several experimental results are presented that demonstrate the efficacy and robustness of the proposed methods.

Keywords: Augmented-Reality, Locomotor training, Spinal-cord injury, Physical Therapy, Rehabilitation, Game, Kinect.

1   Introduction

Locomotor training is an activity based therapy that aims to promote recovery of walking, by activating the neuromuscular system[4]. Locomotor training optimizes task-specific sensory input during intense stepping practice to promote activity-dependent plasticity. While locomotor training was initially developed for persons with spinal cord injuries, it has been recently translated to children and can be used in general with various types of neurologic injuries [14]. In the case of children, during locomotor training, stepping and standing often are practiced on a treadmill for over an hour causing many children to lose motivation and become bored. As attention and focus wane, critical task-specific movements, such as upright trunk posture and reciprocal arm swing, become nearly

---

* This project was in part funded by the NIH/NCATS Clinical and Translational Science Award to the University of Florida UL1 TR000064, and the University of Florida Informatics Institute Seed Fund Award. The authors would like to thank the sponsors and the anonymous volunteers who participated in the pilot study.

C.A. Linte et al. (Eds.): AE-CAI 2014, LNCS 8678, pp. 108–117, 2014.

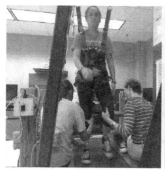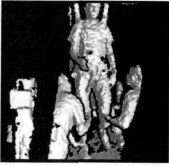

Fig. 1. A picture of our locomotor training environment (left), and the corresponding depth image (right) captured by a depth sensor located on the front of the treadmill.

impossible to evoke. Most importantly, a less intense and effective training session compromises the child's recovery. Incorporation of interactive and engaging video games is an innovative approach to enhance rehabilitation [6,2,5,11,13,7]. Although commercial games have demonstrated therapeutic effects when applied to children with neurological injuries, most games do not consider the specific impairments that are common in children with spinal cord injury and are not designed for use during locomotor training [6,7]. Therefore, our long-term objective is to design and develop an engaging and interactive game that enhances locomotor training for children with neurological injuries.

Our goal is to engage children to perform walking-related movements with their arms and legs in order to play the game. To accomplish this, we use a depth camera to detect and track movement in the unique locomotor training treadmill environment shown in Fig. 1 left. In leterature, there are several examples of methods or applications related to body tracking using depth cameras. A game-based rehabilitation system was presented in [9] using body tracking from RGB-D. Other applications include human detection [15], model-based 3D tracking of hand articulations [10], human pose recognition and tracking of body parts [12], and real-time 3D reconstruction of the articulated human body [3]. A detailed review of RGB-D applications using Microsoft Kinect sensor is presented in [8].

The main challenge in our particular application, which is the main focus of this paper, is that generic body tracking algorithms fail to detect and analyze the patient's body motion due to its close proximity with other objects or human subjects in the locomotor training treadmill environment (see examples in Fig. 5). To overcome this problem we propose a model-free graph-based body segmentation algorithm that detects the arms and legs of the patient. Descriptive motion features are extracted from the segmented regions of the limbs and their movement patterns are analyzed by computing various motion indices that we proposed in this paper to capture the symmetry between the right and left leg kinematics, their pace, and the synchronization of the arm swing with the walking pattern. Several experimental results are presented using real and synthetic data that demonstrate the efficiency of the proposed framework.

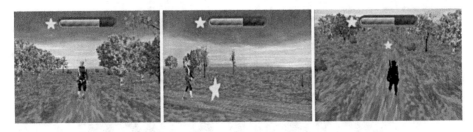

Fig. 2. Screenshots of the developed 3D augmented-reality environment taken from three different orientations to show the front, side, and back of the patient respectively.

2   Methods

In this section, we present our framework for computed-assisted locomotor training using augmented-reality gaming environments (see Fig.2). The framework has two main goals: 1) to enhance the traditional methodologies for physical therapy by exciting kids for walking using gaming technologies, and 2) to compute in real-time several motion-based quantities such as periodicity, synchronization, pace, and others in order to provide the therapist with a quantitative framework for monitoring the progress of a patient, evaluating the effectiveness of therapy, and automatically optimizing the parameters of the therapy.

Motion detection sensors such as infrared depth cameras offer an infrastructure that can facilitate the aforementioned goals and also offer a natural user interface for comunicating with computers without the need of remote controllers or other hand-held or warable electronic devices. Each data frame captured by a digital range camera is a two dimensional array of depth values (i.e., distance between the plane of the sensor and the depicted objects). The depth value of the pixel with coordinates (x, y) on a perticular depth frame is denoted by $d(x, y) \in \mathbb{R}^+$ (see an example of a depth frame in Fig. 1 right).

In the proposed framework, the acquired sequence of depth frames is processed by a graph-based segmentation algorithm that detects the regions of the patient's arms, legs, and torso in the depth images. Descriptive features of the segmented regions are then extracted and employed by motion pattern analysis algorithms, which are described in detail in the following sections.

2.1   Graph-Based Segmentation

Each depth frame is scanned horizontally (row by row) and segmented into line stripes that are smoothly-varing 1-pixel-wide regions defined as

$$\mathcal{L} = \{(x_s, y), \cdots, (x_e, y) : x_s < x_e, \left| \frac{\partial d(x, y)}{\partial x} \right| < \epsilon_1, \left| \frac{\partial^2 d(x, y)}{\partial x^2} \right| < \epsilon_2 \ \forall x \in (x_s, x_e)\}$$

where x_s and x_e denote the start and end pixel coordinates of the line segment. The length of a line segment can be easily computed by $length(\mathcal{L}) = x_e - x_s + 1$.

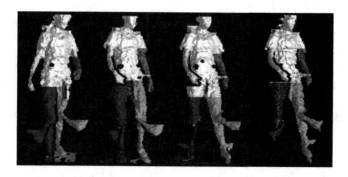

Fig. 3. Representative results of our body segmentation algorithm in different instances during the walking cycle. The generated tree graph is superimposed on the right plate. The partial inclusion of the assistants' arms in the regions of the subject's legs does not affect the estmated motion features as shown in Fig.4, which demonstrates the robustness of the proposed framework to such outliers.

The computed line segments are organized in the form of a directed graph, which is constructed simultaneously with the segmentation of the line segments. In such graph each line segment $\mathcal{L}$ can be connected with line segments in the previous row of pixels that form the set of $parents(\mathcal{L})$ defined as

$$\mathcal{L}' \in parents(\mathcal{L}) \Leftrightarrow \exists(x,y) \in \mathcal{L}, \exists(x,y-1) \in \mathcal{L}' : \left|\frac{\partial d(x,y)}{\partial y}\right| < \epsilon_1. \tag{1}$$

Equivalently, each line segment can be connected with line segments in the next row of pixels by defining the set $children(\mathcal{L})$ as the inverse of Eq. 1 as follows:

$$\mathcal{L}' \in children(\mathcal{L}) \Leftrightarrow \mathcal{L} \in parents(\mathcal{L}'). \tag{2}$$

The graph produced by Eqs. 1 and 2 may contain cycles. To enforce the creation of non-cyclic graphs we define the set $father(\mathcal{L})$ as the subset of $parents(\mathcal{L})$ that contains the largest line segment:

$$father(\mathcal{L}) = \underset{\mathcal{L}' \in parents(\mathcal{L})}{\arg\max} \; length(\mathcal{L}'). \tag{3}$$

The above process segments a given depth frame into several regions that are computed as independent disconnected graphs and typically correspond to different objects in the field of view. In most applications the subject of interest corresponds to the graph with the largest number of pixels, and in general can be easily isolated from the rest of the objects in the scene (see Fig. 3).

Each graph can be further segmented into smoothly varying regions by constructing sets of connected line segments with coherent structural characteristics as follows:

$$S = \{\mathcal{L}_1, \cdots, \mathcal{L}_n : \mathcal{L}_i = father(\mathcal{L}_{i+1}), |children(\mathcal{L}_i)| = 1 \; \forall i \in [i, n-1]\}. \tag{4}$$

The line segments $\mathcal{L}_i$ in Eq. 4 form a sequence of descendants without simblings, which corresponds to a linear graph. The set of segments $\mathcal{S}$ can also be organized into a graph by defining the $father(\mathcal{S})$ and $children(\mathcal{S})$ using the connections defined in $father(\mathcal{L}_1)$ and $children(\mathcal{L}_n)$ respectively. An example of a graph of segments is shown in Fig. 3 (the network of the graph is visualized on the right).

In our application, the regions of the legs and arms of the depicted subjects can be found by performing simple graph searches. More specifically, the legs can be found by searching for the segment with the largest sum of distances from the top of the older ancestor and from the bottom of the youngest descendant. Such distances can be easily computed by accumulating the height of each segment in the corresponding path of the graph given by

$$height(\mathcal{S}) = \max_{\forall(x,y)\in\mathcal{L}_i,\forall\mathcal{L}_i\in\mathcal{S},} y - \min_{\forall(x,y)\in\mathcal{L}_i,\forall\mathcal{L}_i\in\mathcal{S},} y + 1. \tag{5}$$

The left and right children of the solution correspond to the right and left legs respectively. Finally, the left or right arms can be found as the largest right or left children in the graph respectively, which are not already marked as legs. Examples of estimated segments are shown in Fig. 3 with different color-coding.

2.2   Motion Pattern Analysis

After segmenting the regions of the limbs in each depth frame, their motion is analyzed by tracking their motion patterns over time. Various features can be extracted from each segmented region such as the average X, Y, Z coordinate, the medial line, the orientation of the limb, however we found in our experiments that the average Z coordinate of the medial line is descriptive enough to be used in our motion pattern analysis. Hence, four sequences are computed and monitored over time $LL(t)$, $RL(t)$, $LA(t)$, $RA(t)$ that correspond to the average Z coordinate of the medial line of the left leg, right leg, left arm, and right arm regions respectively.

First, each of the sequences is smoothened using a median filter followed by a Gaussian filter to enhance the robustness of our calulations (see example in Fig.4A). Then the local extrema of each sequence are computed as

$$extrema(f(t)) = \begin{cases} 1 & \text{if } t = \arg\max_{t\in N(t)} f(t) \\ -1 & \text{if } t = \arg\min_{t\in N(t)} f(t) \\ 0 & \text{otherwise} \end{cases} , \tag{6}$$

where $N(t)$ is a neighborhood in the time domain centered at t. The size of the neighborhood should be smaller than the duration of each pace to ensure that the extrema of each pace are calculated. Fig. 4B shows Eq. 6 computed from a real data sequence.

The duration between two consecutive same-type extrema (minima or maxima) is given by

$$gap(f(t), v) = \min_{\forall s\geq x:extrema(f(s))=v} s - \max_{\forall s<x:extrema(f(s))=v} s \tag{7}$$

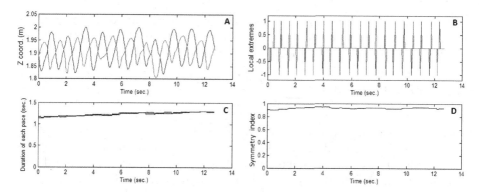

Fig. 4. Experimental results from a real data sequence of 10 paces. A) The estimated z-coordinates of the right (red) and left (blue) leg, B) The time signatures of the estimated local extrema of A, C) The estimated duration of each pace, D) The corresponding symmetry index.

Eq. 7 can be calculated for $LL(t)$ and $RL(t)$ for each type of maxima in order to compute the duration of each pace as a function of time:

$$pace(t) = [gap(LL(t), 1) + gap(LL(t), -1) + gap(RL(t), 1) + gap(RL(t), -1)]/4$$

In a walking pattern with constant speed it is expected that each of the four terms in Eq. 7 gives the same numerical value. However, in practice we compute the average of all four measurements in order to increase the robustness of the overall pace estimator. It should be noted that $pace(t)$ corresponds to the time of a full stride from the time when the recorded signal reaches a local maximum until the time when the same leg's signal reaches the next local maximum (see example in Fig. 4C). The corresponding length of a full stride can be easily computed as $pace(t)/speed$, where $speed$ is the speed of the treadmill, which is a known manually set quantity.

The symmetry of the walking patterns of the two legs as well as their synchronization with the motion of the arms are quantifiable indices that are especially useful for physical therapy. To calculate the level of symmetry of the walking pattern we first need to estimate the mid-point in the time domain between two same-type extrema given by

$$mid(f(t), v) = \left[\min_{\forall s \geq x: extrema(f(s))=v} s + \max_{\forall s < x: extrema(f(s))=v} s \right]/2 \qquad (8)$$

and then compare two sequences $f(t)$ and $g(t)$ by computing the time difference between the extrema of one and the corresponding mid-point of the other as follows:

$$sym(f(t), g(t), v) = 1 - 2 |mid(f(s), v) - s|/pace(s), \qquad (9)$$

where $s = \max_{\forall r < t: extrema(g(r))=v} r$. The largest possible time difference is equal to the duration of half pace, hence the range of Eq. 9 is the interval of real numbers from 0 to 1.

Finally, Eq. 9 considers only one type of extrema of one of the two given sequences. To account for all combinations we compute the symmetry of the walking pattern as the sum of four terms given by

$$symmetry(LL(t), RL(t)) = \sum_{v=-1,1} \frac{sym(LL(t), RL(t), v) + sym(RL(t), LL(t), v)}{4}$$

where $LL(t)$ and $RL(t)$ denote the left and right leg sequences (see Fig. 4D). Similarly, the index that describes the sychnronization between the motion of the legs and the arms can be computed using the arm and leg sequences as follows: $[symmetry(LL(t), LA(t)) + symmetry(RL(t), RA(t))]/2$ (see Fig. 7 left).

2.3   Augmented-Reality Environment

The algorithms presented in Secs. 2.1 and 2.2 were implemented in Java using the J4K (Java for Kinect) Software Development Kit introduced in [3]. The input depth frames are processed in real-time using the proposed graph-based segmentation algorithm and the 3D image of the body of the patient is composed as a textured quadratic mesh by combining the segmented depth image with the corresponding video frame captured by a regular RGB camera.

The 3D image of the body of the patient is visualized within a 3D augmented-reality gaming environment that consists of a randomly generated scene with a walking path. The patient can watch herself walking in this synthesized environment from different 3D views (front, side, and back) that offer visual variability that makes the gaming environment more engaging and easier for the patient to understand the perspective and virtual surroundings (see screenshots in Fig. 2). The environment automatically animates in relation to the speed of the treadmill and new surrounding elements randomly appear as the game progresses.

A scoring system is also used in order to enhance the level of engagement by unlocking new features and environments based on the patient's score. Although in the current version of the game the scoring system is based on the number of items that the user collects from the virtual path, which is proportional to the distance walked, our goal is to introduce adaptive scoring mechanisms that will award good walking patterns based on the calculated symmetry and synchronization of the motion (Sec. 2.2).

3   Experimental Results

In this section, we present several quantitative experimental results obtained by using the proposed framework with real and synthetic data.

Locomotor training typically includes alternate bouts of approximately 5 minutes of treadmill stepping and standing practice to achieve a total of 60-minutes of practice. A team of trainers provide hands-on assistance as well as motivation for the child to step at an age-appropriate/normal speed, maintain an upright trunk posture and normal leg kinematics, and reciprocally swing his or her arms.

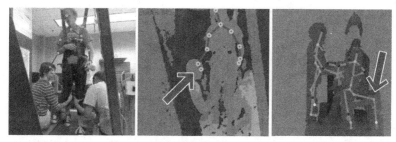

Fig. 5. Typical errors of existing skeleton fitting algorithms caused by the close proximity of the patient with other objects or human subjects in the clinical environment.

To evaluate the feasibility and effectiveness of the proposed framework we organized a pilot study in which we recreated locomotor training sessions in a real clinical setting without employing real patients at this time. During the pilot sessions, depth data were acquired using the PrimeSense^{TM}depth sensor contained in the Microsoft Kinect^{TM}device. The sensor was placed in front of the treadmill and was connected to a 64-bit computer with Intel Core i5 CPU at 2.53GHz and 4GB RAM. The resolution of the depth camera was 320×240 pixels at 25 frames per second and it was calibrated so that it records depth in the range from 0.8m to 4.0m, which is suitable for capturing the patient's motion in our clinical setup. In this hardware setup the proposed algorithms were executed in real-time with average data processing time of 9.9889 ms/frame.

In order to compare our technique with other existing popular methods for body feature extraction from depth frames, we employed the skeleton fitting algorithm provided with the Microsoft Kinect SDK [1]. Our goal was to extract the location and/or orientation of the legs in order to be able to compute the pace and symmetry indices as described in Sec. 2.2. The skeleton fitting algorithm failed to provide full body skeleton for the majority of the depth frames sequences. Instead, upper body tracking was possible, which however does not track the user's legs. The failure of the skeleton fitting algorithm was caused due to the close proximity of the user's body with other objects in our clinical environment. Even in the rare cases in which the algorithm provided output, the obtained skeletons were often erroneous as it is shown in Fig. 5.

In contrast to the Kinect SDK algorithm, our proposed body segmentation algorithm (Sec. 2.1) was able to segment the user's body and provide results for the entire dataset. Fig. 3 shows the segmentation results obtained for four representative frames during the walking cycle. The segmented regions of the arms and legs are color-coded and in the right plate the underlying estimated graph is superimposed. It should be noted that the presence of the assistants' arms in the regions of the subject's legs did not affect our motion analysis because our feature extraction method is robust to such outliers as it is shown in Fig. 4.

Furthermore, we applied the proposed motion analysis framework (Sec. 2.2) to our segmentation results and the computed pace and symmetry indices are presented in the plots of Figs. 4, 6, and 7.

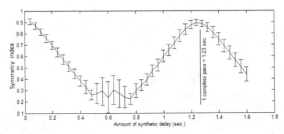

Fig. 6. Plot of the symmetry index versus the amount of synthetic delay introduced in the data sequence of the left leg.

Fig. 4 shows the data sequences extracted from the left and right legs for a period of 10 full strides, and the correspodning extrema, pace, and symmetry index. The red and blue lines correspond to the right and left legs. From the obtained results we can make the following observations: a) the extracted data sequences describe well the walking pattern, b) the pace estimated from the right leg deviates insignificantly from the one of the left leg, which demonstrates the robustness of our model, and c) the calculated symmetry index is very high as expected, which also demonstrates the effectiveness of the proposed index.

More specifically, the average duration of a full stride for a data sample of 60 sec. (Fig. 7) was found to be 1.2350 ± 0.0360 sec. for the left leg and 1.2338 ± 0.0407 sec. for the right leg, with the average for both legs at 1.2344 ± 0.0351 sec. In order to assess the robustness of our algorithm we can multiply these results by the number of acquired frames per second. This will give us an estimated duration of pace of 30.8591 frames with standard deviation of less than a frame (0.8765), which concluively demonstrates that the stability of our estimator reaches the limit of the data acquisition frequency and hence cannot be further improved.

In order to demonstrate the behaviour of the proposed symmetry index in the case of abnormal leg kinematics we introduced various amounts of delays in the sequence of the left leg and for each case we computed the symmetry index. The results are presented in Fig. 6 and show that the symmetry index drops as the amount of delay approaches the half of the pace as expected.

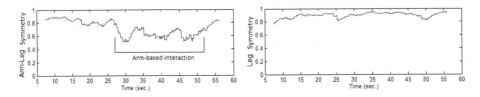

Fig. 7. Plots of the computed arm-leg symmetry (left) and the corresponding leg symmetry (right) from a real data sequence. As expected the motion pattern of the arms has more fluctuations compared to the more coherent symmetry index of the legs.

Finally, Fig. 7 show the arm-leg synchronization (left) in contrast to the symmetry of the leg motion (right). As expected the arm-leg index has higher values when the patient reciprocally swings his or her arms and drops otherwise, for example in the case of hand gestures or other type of arm-based interaction.

4   Conclusion

In this paper a novel framework was presented for locomotor training using an augmented-reality gaming environment, which is remotely controlled with natural user motions detected by a depth camera. The proposed algorithms analyze the motion patterns and compute various descriptive indices that provide the therapists with a quantitative framework for monitoring the progress of the patients. Several experimental results were presented that demonstrated the effectiveness and robustness of our methods. In the future we plan to employ this framework to enhance locomotor training and excite kids for walking.

References

1. Microsoft Kinect SDK, http://www.microsoft.com/enus/kinectforwindows/
2. Adamovich, S., Fluet, G., Tunik, E., Merians, A.: Sensorimotor training in virtual reality: a review. NeuroRehabilitation 25(1), 29–44 (2009)
3. Barmpoutis, A.: Tensor body: Real-time reconstruction of the human body and avatar synthesis from RGB-D. IEEE Trans. on Cybernetics 43(5), 1347–1356 (2013)
4. Behrman, A., Harkema, S.: Locomotor training after human spinal cord injury: a series of case studies. Phys. Ther. 80(7), 688–700 (2000)
5. Bryanton, C., et al.: Feasibility, motivation, and selective motor control: virtual reality compared to conventional home exercise in children with cerebral palsy. Cyberpsychol. Behav. 9(2), 123–128 (2006)
6. Dematteo, C., Greenspoon, D., Levac, D., Harper, J.A., Rubinoff, M.: Evaluating the nintendo wii for assessing return to activity readiness in youth with mild traumatic brain injury. Phys. Occup. Ther. Pediatr. (in print, 2014)
7. Deutsch, J.E., et al.: Use of a low-cost, commercially available gaming console (wii) for rehabilitation of an adolescent with cerebral palsy. Phys. Ther. 88(10) (2008)
8. Han, J., et al.: Enhanced computer vision with Microsoft Kinect sensor: A review. IEEE Transactions on Cybernetics 43(5), 1318–1334 (2013)
9. Lange, B., et al.: Interactive game-based rehabilitation using the Microsoft Kinect. In: IEEE Virtual Reality Workshops, pp. 171–172 (2012)
10. Oikonomidis, I., et al.: Efficient model-based 3d tracking of hand articulations using Kinect. In: Proc. of the British Machine Vision Association Conference (2011)
11. Reid, D.: The influence of virtual reality on playfulness in children with cerebral palsy: a pilot study. Occup. Ther. Int. 11(3), 131–144 (2004)
12. Shotton, J., et al.: Real-time human pose recognition in parts from single depth images. In: IEEE CVPR Conference, pp. 1297–1304 (2011)
13. Walker, M.L., et al.: Virtual reality-enhanced partial body weight-supported treadmill training poststroke: feasibility and effectiveness in 6 subjects. Arch. Phys. Med. Rehabil. 91(1), 115–122 (2010)
14. Willoughby, K.L., et al.: A systematic review of the effectiveness of treadmill training for children with cerebral palsy. Disabil. Rehabil. 31(24), 1971–1979 (2009)
15. Xia, L., et al.: Human detection using depth information by Kinect. In: IEEE Conference on Computer Vision and Pattern Recognition Workshops, pp. 15–22 (2011)

Linear Object Registration of Interventional Tools

Matthew S. Holden and Gabor Fichtinger

Laboratory for Percutaneous Surgery, School of Computing, Queen's University,
Kingston, ON, Canada
{mholden8,gabor}@cs.queensu.ca

Abstract. PURPOSE: Point-set registration for interventional tools requires well-defined points to be present on these tools. In this work, an algorithm is proposed which uses planes, lines, and points for registration when point-set registration is not feasible. METHODS: The proposed algorithm matches points, lines, and planes in each coordinate system, uses invariant features for initial registration, and optimizes the registration iteratively. For validation, simulated data with known ground-truth and real surgical tool registration data using point-set registration as ground-truth were created to evaluate the algorithm's accuracy. RESULTS: The proposed algorithm is equally as accurate as point-set registration, and the difference between the registrations is less than the noise in the tracking system. CONCLUSION: The proposed algorithm is a viable alternative when point-set registration cannot be performed.

Keywords: Registration, Surgical navigation, Coordinate transformations.

1   Introduction and Background

Introduction. Registration is an integral part of all surgical navigation systems, and is used to display interventional tools (including needles, ultrasound probes, phantoms, etc.) and images from multiple modalities in a common navigation space. For example, in surgical simulators with augmented reality, instruments and phantoms must be registered to a common coordinate frame to view them in the augmented reality display [14]. Alternatively, in surgical planning, the plan (and possibly preoperative planning image) must be registered into the same coordinate system as the interventional tools or robots for the procedure [8].

Typical computer-assisted interventions use point-set registration using landmark points identified in both coordinate frames with known correspondence. In most cases, however, landmark points do not naturally occur on physical objects such as interventional tools, robotic devices, or calibration fixtures, and estimating landmarks point positions is insufficiently accurate. Due to engineering constraints, it is more common that an object will have a set of well-defined lines or planes, which could be conveniently and accurately collected and used for registration instead (see, for example, [12] and [15] for instances of such interventional tools).

The objective of this work is to develop and validate a registration algorithm that uses points, lines, and planes (collectively referred to as "linear objects") for registration problems such as those encountered in surgical simulation [14] and planning [8]. The algorithm is designed to provide a convenient alternative when

C.A. Linte et al. (Eds.): AE-CAI 2014, LNCS 8678, pp. 118–127, 2014.
© Springer International Publishing Switzerland 2014

point-set registration is infeasible. Such an algorithm should work for any set of linear objects that uniquely defines the registration and should be guaranteed to converge an approximately optimal solution in polynomial time. Additionally, the algorithm should work even when one set of linear objects is a permuted subset of the other.

Although the proposed algorithm is validated by registering man-made objects with linear features that can be localized with a pointing device, the algorithm has further applications in image registration, which could be performed using linear features extracted from images of interventional tools (which has previously been shown to be a fruitful endeavour [10]).

Background. Many point-set registration methods have been proposed for points with unknown correspondence based on Besl and McKay's [1] iterative closest point algorithm. Several methods proposed to improve convergence to the global optimum include: using symmetry to achieve a better initial guess [6], "Lipschitzizing" the error function [9], or using a Levenberg-Marquardt method [4]. Regardless, a global optimum can only be guaranteed with great computational expense.

Alternative approaches use invariant features in both coordinate frames to find the correspondences and then apply a closed-form solution. Thirion [13] used the extreme points of the dataset to determine correspondences. Xiao *et al.* [16] matched surface properties of local point clouds to determine correspondences. Similar feature extraction techniques are also used in many image registration algorithms. Unfortunately, most of these methods rely on having a complete set of points collected in both coordinate frames, which is unavailable in many situations.

Several works provide algorithms which satisfy some criteria for solving the problem outlined above. Jain *et al.* [7] use points, lines, and ellipses for registration of C-arm images. Their work, however, uses specific features of C-arm imaging and is not guaranteed to converge. Lee *et al.* [8] also perform image registration using fiducial lines and their cross-sectional images. Their work does not consider the case of fiducial planes or points, and thus, does not apply in all scenarios examined here.

The work of Meyer *et al.* [10] used a combination of points, lines, and planes (i.e. linear objects) with known correspondence for image registration. For each linear object, they calculate the projection of the centroid onto it and the direction vector from the projection to the centroid. The coordinate frames are registered using these points with known correspondence. Our proposed algorithm improves upon their algorithm by automatically determining linear object correspondence, not requiring points to define the centroid, and offering an iterative method for convergence.

Olsson *et al.* [11] provide a branch and bound method for registering a set of points to their corresponding points, lines, and planes. They provide an algorithm which is guaranteed to converge to the optimal solution for any configuration. Though our proposed algorithm only guarantees convergence to a near globally optimal solution, it has the advantage of being polynomial time, rather than exponential time.

Overall, the proposed algorithm extends previous work [10] by providing automatic linear object matching, solutions to a wider range of configurations, and offering an iterative convergence method. In contrast to [11], the proposed algorithm runs in polynomial time. Furthermore, an open-source implementation of the proposed algorithm is provided through the SlicerIGT (www.slicerigt.org) extension for 3D slicer (www.slicer.org), thus providing an accessible medical registration tool.

2   Methods

2.1   Linear Object Registration Algorithm (LORA)

Point-to-Point, Line-to-Line, Plane-to-Plane Registration. This represents the most important component of the proposed algorithm: a method for simultaneously registering points to points, lines to lines, and planes to planes. The solution is guaranteed to be approximately optimal and the algorithm runs in polynomial time.

To this end, the centroid of a set of linear objects $\overline{X}$ is defined as the point for which the sum of squared distances to all linear objects X is minimized.

$$\overline{X} = \arg \min_{\bar{x} \in R^3} \left[\sum_{x \in X} D^2(\bar{x}, x) \right]$$

(1)

In practice, the centroid can be calculated by finding the least-squares solution $\overline{X}$ to the below equation, where each linear object has some point $\vec{b}$ that lies on it and some orthonormal basis $\vec{n}$ to its orthogonal subspace.

$$\begin{bmatrix} \vec{n}_1^T \\ ... \\ \vec{n}_m^T \end{bmatrix} \overline{X} = \begin{bmatrix} \vec{n}_1^T \vec{b}_1 \\ ... \\ \vec{n}_m^T \vec{b}_m \end{bmatrix}$$

(2)

The method for simultaneously registering points to points, lines to lines, and planes to planes follows as below, assuming registration of linear objects in coordinate frame A to linear objects in coordinate frame B.

1. Calculate the linear object centroid for linear objects in frame A and the linear object centroid for linear objects in frame B.
2. In both coordinate frames, translate the linear objects such that the centroid lies at the origin of the coordinate frame.
3. For each coordinate frame, respectively, denote $\vec{y}_A$ and $\vec{y}_B$ as the set of closest points on each linear object to the origin.
4. For each line and plane, add the direction or normal vector to the set $\vec{y}_A$ or $\vec{y}_B$ as applicable.
5. Calculate the point-set registration between the sets $\vec{y}_A$ and $\vec{y}_B$.

Linear Object Matching. Automatically determining correspondence is an important component of the proposed algorithm in terms of usability. Ideally, intrinsic features that are invariant between the two sets of linear objects could be used. By considering the counterexample of registering three equidistant points (for which the registration is unique given correspondence), however, it can readily be seen that any matching will produce a solution with the same fiducial registration error. Thus, some external feature must be used to determine linear object correspondence.

The chosen external feature is a set of fiducials which have invariance between the two coordinate frames, which shall be called "references". These are not used for registration directly, but are used to determine the correspondence between linear objects. These references need not be collected with high accuracy, however, since they are not used directly for registration. A linear object's signature is defined as the vector of distances to the set of references $R = \{r_1, ..., r_K\}$.

$$signature(L) = [D(L, r_1), ..., D(L, r_K)] \tag{3}$$

Linear objects in the two coordinate frames can be matched by comparing their signatures. Linear objects whose signatures cannot be matched (to within some threshold) are discarded. The matching threshold is calculated as the product of the noise associated with collecting the linear objects and the number of references.

Reconstructing Linear Objects from Point Sets. In practice, linear objects may be collected discretely. Thus, rather than points, lines, and planes, one set of linear objects may look like a set of points clustered about points, lying on lines, and/or lying on planes (see Fig. 1). It is assumed that point-sets are delineated such that each subset describes precisely one linear object. Then, the principal component analysis

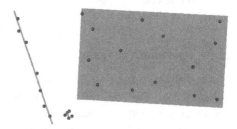

Fig. 1. Illustration of a point, line, and plane (blue) reconstructed from a set of points (red)

for each subset may be calculated, where the eigenvectors associated with non-zero eigenvalues represent direction vectors on the linear object. These derived linear objects may be subsequently used for linear object registration.

Moreover, these initial points used to extract the linear objects may be used to improve the registration result. Given an initial registration and known correspondence, the registration between a set of linear objects in coordinate frame A, and a set of points $b = \{b_1, ..., b_n\}$ in frame B can be calculated as follows.

1. Transform each point b_i in coordinate frame B by the current transform T.
2. For each transformed point Tb_i, find the closest point a_i on its corresponding linear object in coordinate frame A.
3. Shift the sets a_i and b_i such that their centroids $\bar{a}$ and $\bar{b}$ lie at the origin.
4. Calculate the pure rotational registration R between a_i and b_i.
5. Recalculate the current transform. Its rotation is R and its translation is $\bar{a} - R\bar{b}$.
6. Iterate until some convergence criteria is met (for example, the change in fiducial registration error is below some threshold).

Linear Object Registration Algorithm. In summary, LORA proceeds as follows.

1. Reconstruct linear objects from collected points, as applicable.
2. Compute linear object correspondences using references.
3. Perform point-to-point, line-to-line, and plane-to-plane registration.
4. Use the result from step 3 as an initial transform in an iterative point-set to linear object registration.

Step 3, being the key step in the algorithm, offers a closed-form solution to the point-to-point, line-to-line, and plane-to-plane registration. It produces an exact solution to a finite version of the linear object registration problem which is globally optimal for the inifinite version in the case of no noise. This means that in practical cases where there is noise, step 3 produces an approximate solution. Step 4 is guaranteed to converge to a local minimum (by extension of the proof of convergence from [1]), so the entire solution is guaranteed to be approximate.

2.2   Algorithm Validation

Simulated Data. As an initial form of validation, LORA's feasibility was tested on simulated data. The objective of the simulation was to generate random linear objects and to create random points on these linear objects, transformed by a known transformation matrix. Since the ground-truth transformation is known, the algorithm's accuracy can be readily evaluated.

A random transformation matrix can be generated by generating a random rotation and a random translation separately and combining the results. To generate a random rotation R, any matrix M with randomly generated elements and its singular value decomposition may be used.

$$M = UDV^T \tag{4}$$

$$R = UV^T \tag{5}$$

The translation $\vec{d}$ is generated by picking each component randomly.

1. Generate a random number of each type of linear object (with random position and orientation) in coordinate frame A. Generate four references with random position in coordinate frame A.
2. For each linear object L in coordinate frame A, generate a set of random points $a = \{a_1, ..., a_n\}$ lying on L.
3. Generate a random transformation matrix T (by above described method).
4. Apply the random transformation matrix to each random point Ta_i, and add Gaussian noise in each dimension.

This algorithm generates random linear objects in coordinate frame A and simulates point collection in frame B on the linear objects. Thus, this simulated data can be used to test the feasibilty of LORA by comparing its result to the ground-truth.

Real Data. As interventional tools in the general sense, three previously developed surgical navigation phantoms were used for validation of LORA: an fCal ultrasound calibration phantom (Fig. 2a) [3], a lumbar spine phantom (Fig. 2b) [14], and a LEGO® ultrasound calibration phantom (Fig. 2c) [15]. Though these are not traditional interventional tools, the validation results apply equally to registration of tracked tools such as ultrasound probes or scalpels. The objective was to find the transformation between the phantoms' sensor's coordinate frame and the navigation system coordinate frame. This form of registration is required in surgical simulators to display all the objects in a common navigation space [14].

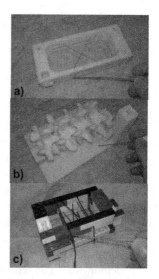

For each phantom, the set of linear objects in the phantom coordinate frame was defined. Both ultrasound calibration phantoms had a box-like exterior. Each face of this box was defined as a linear object. The lumbar spine phantom sits on a rectangular prism base. Each face of the base was defined as a linear object. Also, the vertebrae are mounted on a block that is attached to the base. The lines where this block attaches to the base were defined as linear objects.

Fig. 2. Photographs of a user collecting points on a) fCal [3], b) lumbar spine [14], and c) LEGO® [15] phantoms

The fCal and lumbar spine phantoms already had points machined on them for point-set registration purposes. Using these points, point-set registration for each phantom was performed and used as ground-truth against which LORA was compared. The LEGO® phantom did not have points machined on it, so LORA was validated by comparing target registration errors and point reconstruction accuracies [2] from point-set registration (using approximate fiducial positions) and LORA.

For validation, all linear objects defined on each phantom were used, and two reference points were chosen from the set of points used for point-set registration. A 0.9mm stylus, tracked using the Ascension TrakStar electromagnetic tracking system (www.ascension-tech.com), was used to collect points on each linear object. The stylus was placed with its tip at each point, the stylus tip was traced back and forth along each line, and the stylus tip was slid over the entire extent of each plane. All data was collected, annotated, and saved using 3D Slicer (www.slicer.org).

3   Results

To compare two transformations, the translational error metric was calculated as the norm of the difference between the two translations:

$$E_{TRANSLATION} = \left| \vec{d}_1 - \vec{d}_2 \right| \tag{6}$$

The rotational error metric was calculated as the angle (from the axis-angle representation) of rotation of the quotient of the two rotation matrices:

$$E_{ROTATION} = \arccos\left(\left(tr\left(R_1^{-1}R_2\right)-1\right)/2\right) \qquad (7)$$

Simulated Data. To demonstrate the robustness of LORA in simulation, the average translational and rotational error over fifty trials associated with the registration (compared to the ground-truth) is plotted for varying levels of Gaussian noise (Fig. 3). Most importantly, the error increases linearly with the noise, demonstrating the robustness of LORA.

The Ascension TrakStar electromagnetic tracking system (www.ascension-tech.com) reports 1.4mm root-mean-square tracking accuracy. Using this level of simulated noise, the algorithm exhibits 0.085° rotational error and 0.21mm translational error.

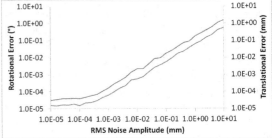

Fig. 3. Plot of translational error (red) and rotational error (blue) in the calculated transformation as a function of root-mean-square noise in the simulated data

To demonstrate the required number of references, simulated data was generated using varying number of references. The linear object matching was successful over 90% of the time when there was one reference. For two or more references, matching was successful in every simulation trial (up to 10.0mm of root-mean-square noise), indicating that two references are sufficient for practical linear object registration.

Real Data. For all three phantoms, the linear object registration had smaller average root-mean-square error than the traditional point-set registration (1.22mm vs. 2.13mm for the fCal ultrasound calibration phantom, 1.14mm vs. 1.33mm for the lumbar spine phantom, and 0.45mm vs. 0.53mm for the LEGO® phantom).

The error between the ground-truth (calculated as the mean transform from the point-set registration) and the transformation calculated using LORA is displayed in Table 1. The variability in the results produced by each algorithm is shown in Table 2. This provides a measure of each algorithm's precision.

Translational variability for the lumbar spine phantom was the only significantly different reported variability (two-tailed t-test, $p = 0.003$) between the two algorithms.

Table 1. Error metrics for linear object registration using the fCal and lumbar spine phantoms. Error is calculated as the mean difference between the linear object registrations and the mean point-set registration. The rotational and translational errors are averaged over all registrations.

Metric	fCal Phantom	Lumbar Spine Phantom
Rotational Error (°)	1.49	0.76
Translational Error (mm)	0.74	1.15

The target registration errors and point reconstruction accuracies for the LEGO® phantom are shown for each algorithm in Table 3. The point reconstruction accuracies are so large due to noise in the electromagnetic tracking system; however, LORA still produces significantly better accuracies than point-set registration. Both metrics are significantly smaller for LORA (by two-tailed t-test), with medium-large effect size using Cohen's d statistic ($p = 0.005$, effect size 0.57 for target registration error; $p < 0.001$, effect size 0.68 for point reconstruction accuracy).

Table 2. Rotational and translational precisions for each registration algorithm for the fCal and lumbar spine phantoms. The precision is calculated as the mean difference between each registration and the mean registration.

fCal Phantom		
Metric	Point-Set Registration	Linear Object Registration
Rotational Precision (°)	0.46	0.43
Translational Precision (mm)	0.45	0.37
Lumbar Spine Phantom		
Metric	Point-Set Registration	Linear Object Registration
Rotational Precision (°)	0.29	0.42
Translational Precision (mm)	0.35	0.76

Table 3. Target registration error and point reconstruction accuracy for point-set registation and LORA on the LEGO® ultrasound calibration phantom

Target Registration Error		
Metric	Point-Set Registration	Linear Object Registration
Mean (mm)	1.34	1.18
Standard Deviation (mm)	0.31	0.22
Point Reconstruction Accuracy		
Metric	Point-Set Registration	Linear Object Registration
Mean (mm)	3.98	3.46
Standard Deviation (mm)	0.64	0.80

For our current Matlab implementation, LORA took on average 34s with 9,816 collected points for the fCal phantom, 71s with 11,969 collected points for the lumbar spine phantom, and 57s with 10,380 collected points for the LEGO® phantom. For surgical simulation and planning, registrations are typically performed offline; thus, this temporal performance is adequate for practical use. In all instances, point-set registration took less than 1s to complete, but uses fewer than ten points. These performance results contrast with results from Olsson et al. [11], which took up to 30s with fewer than twenty collected points. With our dataset, which contains up to 10,000 collected points per registration, their algorithm could take impractically long.

4   Discussion and Conclusion

Fitzpatrick et al. [5] prove that target registration error decreases with distance to the centroid and with larger fiducial configurations. This implies that linear objects should encompass relevant structures, and points should be collected on the entirety of linear objects. For example, for both ultrasound calibration phantoms, the linear objects should encompass the calibration wires, and for the lumbar spine phantom, the linear objects should encompass the intervertebral spaces. Linear objects are usually completely defined by the surgical tool itself, however, and should not need to be modified for registration. The results from the simulated data using random geometry suggest that LORA is robust to the arrangement of linear objects.

Additionally, Fitzpatrick *et al.* [5], show that target registration error also decreases as more points are collected for registration. Thus, the number and range of collected points on each linear object should be maximized to improve the accuracy of LORA.

Some sets of linear objects are insufficient to specify the transformation between the tool sensor coordinate frame and the surgical tool coordinate frame completely. Importantly, LORA has the property that it will calculate the transformation between the two coordinate frames for any sufficient set of linear objects.

One less robust aspect of LORA is matching. Although simulated results show that two references is sufficient, it can be inconvenient to collect many references. One possibility is to enforce that the user manually match the linear objects. Alternatively, geometrical constraints on the defined references and linear objects could be enforced to ensure unambiguous matching.

The results reported here are strictly from surgical tool registration applications, however, the algorithm extends to related applications, for which limited further validation is required. Other applications for LORA include image registration. LORA offers a general method to register imaged points, lines, or planes with interventional tools including robots, or Z-frame and N-wire phantoms, without requiring development of a new registration algorithm. Validation of the proposed algorithm for surgical planing and image registration is a clinical setting is required.

Of course, not all interventional tools consist of well-defined linear objects. LORA could be extended to registration of any parametrically defined surfaces or curves. This, however, may be problematic since parametrically defined objects do not necessarily have the properties of linear objects used by LORA.

The proposed algorithm has been made available through the open-source SlicerIGT (www.slicerigt.org) extension for 3D Slicer (www.slicer.org). This provides a convenient interface for users to collect linear objects and use LORA. Further usability and temporal performance studies for the module are planned.

In conclusion, an algorithm (LORA) for surgical tool registration using linear objects has been developed, implemented, and validated. The algorithm does not impose the constraint of well-defined points that point-set registration algorithms impose. The algorithm works on a principle of extracting corresponding points from the linear objects in the two coordinate frames using geometric invariants and performing point-set registration on these, following by an iterative algorithm to converge to an optimum, which is guaranteed to be close to the global optimum. This algorithm was validated on simulated data by showing that the error in the registration increases linearly with noise in the data. The algorithm was validated using three different surgical navigation objects. Results showed that LORA performs practically identically to ground-truth point-set registration and it demonstrates more favorable registration error metrics while it is significantly more convenient to apply in practice.

References

1. Besl, P.J., McKay, N.D.: A Method for Registration of 3D Shapes. IEEE Transactions on Pattern Analysis and Machine Intelligence 14, 239–256 (1992)
2. Carbajal, G., et al.: Improving N-wire phantom-based freehand ultrasound calibration. International Journal of Computer Assisted Radiology and Surgery 8, 1063–1072 (2013)
3. Chen, T.K., et al.: A Real-Time Freehand Ultrasound Calibration System with Automatic Accuracy Feedback and Control. Ultrasound in Medicine & Biology 35(1), 79–93 (2009)
4. Fitzgibbon, A.W.: Robust Registration of 2D and 3D Point Sets. Image and Vision Computing 21, 1145–1153 (2003)
5. Fitzpatrick, J.M., West, J.B., Maurer, C.R.: Predicting Error in Rigid-Body Registration. IEEE Transactions on Medical Imaging 17, 694–702 (1998)
6. Foroughi, P., Taylor, R., Fichtinger, G.: Revisited Initialization for 3D Bone Registration. In: Proceedings of SPIE (2008)
7. Jain, A.K., et al.: FTRAC - A robust fluoroscopic tracking fiducial. Medical Physics 32(10), 3185–3198 (2005)
8. Lee, S., Fichtinger, G., Chirikjian, G.S.: Numerical algorithms for spatial registration of line fiducial from cross-sectional images. Medical Physics 29(8), 1881–1891 (2002)
9. Li, H., Hartley, R.: The 3D-3D Registration Problem Revisited. In: IEEE International Conference on Computer Vision (2007)
10. Meyer, C.R., et al.: Simultaneous Usage of Homologous Points, Lines, and Planes for Optimal 3D, Linear Registration of Multimodality Imaging Data. IEEE Transactions on Medical Imaging 14, 1–11 (1995)
11. Olsson, C., Kahl, F., Oskarsson, M.: Branch-and-Bound Methods for Euclidean Registration Problems. IEEE Transactions on Pattern Analysis and Machine Intelligence 31(5), 783–794 (2009)
12. Shamir, R., Freiman, M., Joskowicz, L., Shoham, M., Zehavi, E., Shoshan, Y.: Robot-Assisted Image-Guided Targeting for Minimally Invasive Neurosurgery: Planning, Registration, and In-vitro Experiment. In: Duncan, J.S., Gerig, G., et al. (eds.) MICCAI 2005. LNCS, vol. 3750, pp. 131–138. Springer, Heidelberg (2005)
13. Thirion, J.P.: Extremal Points: Definition and Application to 3D Image Registration. In: Proceedings of the IEEE Computer Society Conference on Computer Vision and Pattern Recognition (1994)
14. Ungi, T., et al.: Perk Tutor: An open-source training platform for ultrasound-guided needle insertions. IEEE Transactions on Biomedical Engineering 59(12), 3475–3481 (2012)
15. Walsh, R., et al.: Design of a tracked ultrasound calibration made of LEGO bricks. In: SPIE Medical Imaging (2014)
16. Xiao, G., Ong, S.H., Foong, K.W.C.: Efficient Partial-Surface Registration for 3D Objects. Computer Vision and Image Understanding 98, 271–293 (2005)

Augmented Reality-Enhanced Endoscopic Images for Annuloplasty Ring Sizing

Sandy Engelhardt[1], Raffaele De Simone[2], Norbert Zimmermann[2],
Sameer Al-Maisary[2], Diana Nabers[1], Matthias Karck[2], Hans-Peter Meinzer[1],
and Ivo Wolf[1,3]

[1] Div. of Medical and Biological Informatics,
German Cancer Research Center (DKFZ), Heidelberg, Germany
[2] Department of Cardiac Surgery, University of Heidelberg, Heidelberg, Germany
[3] Institute for Medical Informatics, Mannheim University of Applied Sciences,
Mannheim, Germany

Abstract. Mitral valve annuloplasty is done in patients with mitral
valve insufficiency in order to stabilize, remodel or downsize the often
symmetrical or asymmetrical dilated annulus by stitching a prosthetic
ring on this anatomical structure. Prosthetic rings are available in different shapes and sizes. State-of-the-art intraoperative sizing techniques
for determination of the appropriate ring prosthesis are ambiguous and
highly depend on the surgeon's expertise. We propose a new augmented
reality environment for visualizing the prosthetic ring *in-situ* on endoscopic images and therefore aid in ring selection. The superimposed ring
gives quantitative information and visual cues allowing to compare the
selected ring prosthesis with the patient's annulus. Furthermore, it helps
in determination of regions where an asymmetrical dilatation can be observed. Our method identifies 2D points on the endoscopic images by
detecting the entry points of the mattress sutures into the annular tissue
for ring fixation. 3D shape information of the annulus are obtained from
ultrasound images of the patient. The pose estimation problem of the
3D annulus model is solved using an adapted iterative closest point algorithm. Neither additional hardware nor placement of artificial fiducial
markers are required by the proposed approach.

Keywords: Augmented Reality, Endoscopy, Surgical Suture Detection,
Mitral Valve Annuloplasty, Minimal-Invasive Valve Reconstruction.

1 Introduction

The mitral valve (MV) is a complex apparatus consisting of the annulus, the two
leaflets, chordae tendineae, and papillary muscles, which are required to act together throughout the cardiac cycle. The fibromuscular annulus is a ring-shaped
structure, which anchors the anterior and posterior leaflets. In degenerative,
myxomatous or ischemic diseases, the annulus is prone to symmetric or asymmetric dilation, which can provoke dysfunctions, resulting in MV stenosis or
regurgitation. Both conditions reduce the pumping function of the heart, which
may cause life-threatening conditions that demand for valve surgery.

C.A. Linte et al. (Eds.): AE-CAI 2014, LNCS 8678, pp. 128–137, 2014.
© Springer International Publishing Switzerland 2014

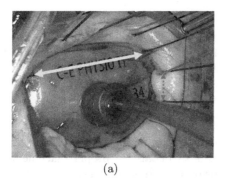
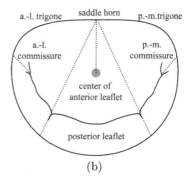

(a)   (b)

Fig. 1. (a) Example of conventional sizing. The yellow arrowheads point to notches on the sizing instrument, which have to be aligned with the commissural points. Each green, dashed arrowhead points to the entry point of a mattress sutures following the recommendations of Carpentier (see section 1.2). (b) Illustration of the MV morphology. The saddle horn is the closest point on the annulus from the center of the anterior leaflet. a.-l.=anterolateral, p.-m.=posteromedial.

1.1 Mitral Valve Reconstrunction

For patients without pathological findings in the MV tissue, reconstruction techniques can be applied instead of a valve replacement. An important surgical technique of MV reconstruction is the annuloplasty: a suitable commercially available ring prosthesis is implanted on the native annulus in order to stabilize or remodel its size and shape. Choosing the proper ring type has been described as critical step during the operation [7]. If the ring is too narrow, functional mitral stenosis, systolic anterior motion or even ring dehiscence might occur. If the ring is oversized, regurgitation might reappear.

The traditional method for ring selection is the intraoperative so-called *sizing* procedure. The size of the annulus is assessed by the surgeon using a *sizer* instrument, which is a flat template that is placed on the MV (see figure 1(a)). Different types of sizers with notches at the commissural or trigonal points are provided by the manufactures and various sizing strategies are described in the literature [1][2]. The opinions on how to select the appropriate ring shape and size vary significantly among surgeons and often appear arbitrary and without scientific justification. Bothe et al. [1] describe inconsistencies in the application of ring sizers that make surgical success depend more on experience and personal judgement than on objective measurements: the dimensions of the sizers may not match the dimensions of their respective annuloplasty ring and the dimensions of the sizers from different manufacturers differ although ring dimensions are identical. Thus, an operator-independent and less experience-based sizing strategy may be helpful to optimize surgical success and patient outcome [1].

In this paper, we propose a technique for *in-situ* visualization of the pre-segmented annulus and the chosen ring using Augmented Reality (AR). The ring is superimposed on endoscopic images acquired during minimal invasive mitral valve reconstructions, providing a preview of the implantation result. This system can have additional future applications for example by visualizing predicted stress levels acting on the implanted ring prosthesis. To the best of our knowledge, this is the first AR system for annuloplasty ring sizing using endoscopic images.

1.2 Recommendations for Annuloplasty Ring Implantation

According to Alain Carpentier, pioneering surgeon in the field of mitral valve reconstruction, the ring implantation meets two goals [3]: proper placement of the sutures (1) within the annulus fibrosus to avoid ring dehiscence, and (2) into the prosthetic ring to avoid annuluar distortion. These recommendations are followed by surgeons worldwide. Considering the first objective, ring implantation is achieved by placing a series of 12 to 15 mattress sutures through the mitral annulus (see figure 1(a)). The width of each suture is guided by the curvature of the 3/8 needle. It must not be smaller than 8 mm to avoid pulling the suture through the annulus, and no larger than 1 cm to prevent distortion of the anterior leaflet. The intervall between the mattress sutures should not exceed 2 mm. In case of an asymmetrical dilatation, more sutures should be placed in the dilated part. White and green sutures should be placed alternately to avoid confusion between the free suture ends. Considering the ring alignment, the two commissural sutures should be passed through the selected ring at the exact corresponding positions. This is an essential precaution to avoid malpositioning of the ring and therefore a distortion of the annulus. The posterior midpoint of the ring should be aligned to the saddle horn. The sutures are then evenly and equally passed from the annulus through the corresponding parts of the ring.

2   Methods

The AR system has been implemented as a plugin of the free open-source *Medical Imaging Interaction Toolkit* (MITK) [9]. The choice of methods and the workflow was designed that neither additional hardware (e.g., a tracking system), nor artificial fiducials are required. Instead, we take the well-defined organization of the sutures (see section 1.2) as given fiducials in the scene.

Intraoperative endoscopic video (using a monoscopic HD endoscope by Karl Storz, Tuttlingen, Germany) and 3D+t transesophageal echocardiography (TEE)-ultrasound data from a patient with MV insufficiency who underwent minimal-invasive mitral valve reconstruction (without robotic support) were collected. The annulus was interactively segmented using the *MITK Mitralyzer* [5] from a systolic time step of the 3D+t TEE ultrasound data. This 3D annulus model is used for 3D pose estimation. Fourteen commercially available rigid annuloplasty rings were digitized by computer tomography and virtual models have been produced. Intrinsic camera parameters were determined using the OpenCV implementation of Zhang's method [14]. A short scene (571 frames, 1920 × 1080 pixel) after the placement of the sutures were extracted from the video. The upper image in figure 2 shows an exemplary frame. Besides the brighter valve tissue and the white

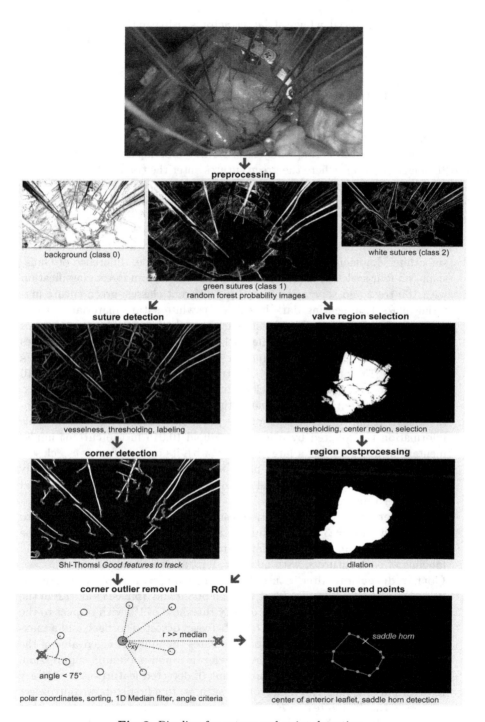

Fig. 2. Pipeline for suture end point detection

and green suture material, a huge atrial retractor is visible in the endoscopic video sequence to allow for an optimal exposure of the valve. The surrounding tissue is the reddish-yellow epicardium.

2.1   Suture Detection on Endoscopic Images

Our method is based on detecting green nonabsorbable 2-0 polyester sutures (Ethibond Excel™, Ethicon Endo-Surgery, USA) on endoscopic images. This braided suture material is frequently used for MV annuloplasty. Of interest are the 2D image positions where the green sutures enter the tissue. Our solution to this problem is to exploit different visual cues such as color and shape information. The pipeline is depicted in figure 2 and described in the following.

- **Classification** For preprocessing of the RGB frames, we chose a learning-based approach using on each RGB channel four feature types (Gaussian smoothing, Laplacian of Gaussian, gradient magnitude, difference of Gaussians) on four scales ($\sigma \in \{0.7, 1.0, 1.6, 3.5\}$) in a random forest classification with 100 trees and separation into three different classes: green suture material (class 1, appearing dark in figure 2), white suture material (class 2, appearing reddish due to blood) and background (class 0). The green sutures (class 1) distinguish well from the background and from the white sutures and is used in the pipeline for further postprocessing. We used the *ilastik toolkit* v0.5 [13] for this purpose. For training, we marked 10 green and 10 white sutures and parts of the background with the annotation tool of ilastik.
- **MV region selection** The tissue of the MV appears as a almost homogenous dark region in the center of the probability image for class 1. This information is exploited by using a threshold (0.015 in the current implementation) and selecting a large region R with its center of mass c_{xy} closest to the center of the image. In a next step, the region R is morphologically dilated to region R_d with a kernel of size 18 to include proximal sutures and to produce a mask.
- **Suture detection** On classification result 1, the 2D vesselness filter by Sato et al. [11] with $\sigma = 3$ and a radius pyramid of 3,4,..,7 is applied, since the sutures have a tubular shape similar to vessels. Further thresholding and labeling of each suture s_l with label $l = 1, ..., n$ are carried out.
- **Corner detection** After suture detection, strong corners p_{xy}^l are detected using the *Good Features To Track* method of Shi and Tomasi et al. [12] in the OpenCV implementation (with a quality threshold of 1% with respect to the best corner, a minimum distance of 10 between detected corners, and a maximum of 200 corners). This method calculates the minimal eigenvalue of the covariance matrix of derivatives and performs a non-maximum suppression.
- **Corner outlier removal** Postprocessing of detected features is neccessary to determine the final end points of the sutures. In a first step, we only select corners in the dilated region R_d. For each suture s_l, select the corner $\tilde{p}_{xy}^l$ that has the smallest Euclidean distance to the center of mass c_{xy} of the region R. The corners $\tilde{p}_{xy}^l$ are converted to polar coordinates r, ϕ with a coordinate

system centered at c_{xy}, then $\tilde{p}^l_{r,\phi}$ are sorted in accending order according to the angle ϕ. Now, a 1D-median filter of size 5 is applied to $r(\tilde{p}^l_{r,\phi})$. $\tilde{p}^l_{r,\phi}$ with large deviation from the median radius are excluded. Furthermore, an angle criteria is applied to the set of remaining $\tilde{p}^l_{r,\phi}$, allowing only neighboring corners to be connected by lines that have an inner angle of $> 75°$ (see figure 2 bottom left).

- **Saddle horn detection** A specific anatomical landmark, the saddle horn, has been identified on the septal portion of the mitral annulus (see figure 1(b)) in order to have a good first guess in terms of the position of the 3D annulus model for 3D pose estimation. The fast Euclidean distance transform of binary images by Maurer et al. [8] has been applied to the region R. The distance transform results in the largest negative value in the center of the anterior leaflet. The centroid from the leaflet center region is computed and the point on the annulus with the shortest distance to the centroid is selected as saddle horn.

2.2   3D Pose Estimation

Given the 2D positions of the surgical suture entry points, we estimate the corresponding 3D pose of the presegmented annulus model. By pose we mean the transformation needed to map an object model from its inherent coordinate system into agreement with sensory data such as image data [10], in our case the endoscopic video data. The projection rays from the calibrated camera through the 2D points on the image plane are reconstructed. The algorithm is based on the idea that the position of the corresponding 3D points on the ring model are restricted by the reconstructed rays. Tentative correspondences between the 3D points on each ray closest to a point on the 3D object contour are established. Next, the rigid transform between the object contour points and the points on the ray are computed that gives the best fit mapping one onto the other in a least squares sense. The pose estimation algorithm can be summarized as follows:

(a) **Ray Reconstruction** Reconstruction of projection rays from the center of the camera through the 2D suture end points on the image plane
(b) **Initial Pose** Initial positioning of 3D annulus model in the arithmetic mean of the rays; rotation of 3D annulus model to align with the saddle horn
(c) **Correspondences** The closest points of each projection ray to a point on the 3D annulus model are taken as tentative correspondences
(d) **Rigid Transformation** Estimation of the pose of the 3D annulus model using this correspondence set as input for Horns method [6]
(e) **Error Calculation** goto (c), if mean Euclidean distance between the tentative corresponding 3D points is > 1 mm or number of iterations is < 1000.

Due to the oval shape of the annulus and the perspective distortion, the correct rotation of the annulus model about the axis normal to the annular plane is hard to estimate by an unrestriced pose estimation algorithm. Therefore, we give a higher weight to the known correspondence of the saddle horn by inserting the

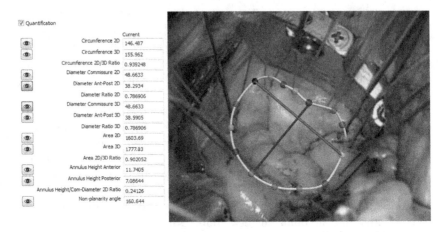

☑ Quantification

		Current
👁	Circumference 2D	146.487
👁	Circumference 3D	155.962
	Circumference 2D/3D Ratio	0.939248
👁	Diameter Commissure 2D	48.6633
👁	Diameter Ant-Post 2D	38.2934
	Diameter Ratio 2D	0.786906
👁	Diameter Commissure 3D	48.6633
👁	Diameter Ant-Post 3D	38.5905
	Diameter Ratio 3D	0.786906
👁	Area 2D	1603.69
👁	Area 3D	1777.83
	Area 2D/3D Ratio	0.902052
👁	Annulus Height Anterior	11.7405
👁	Annulus Height Posterior	7.08644
	Annulus Height/Com-Diameter 2D Ratio	0.24126
👁	Non-planarity angle	160.644

Fig. 3. Automatic quantifications and result of 3D pose estimation of the presegmented mitral annulus model fitted to the suture end points. The upper blue sphere indicates the saddle horn.

correspondence five times into the set of correspondences. Thus, transformations away from this point are highly penalized during the least squares solution.

2.3 Augmented Reality Environment

When the final pose has been found, the 3D annulus model is reprojected onto the image plane using the intrinsic parameters of the calibrated camera and superimposed on the endoscopic image, giving a visual impression about the quality of pose estimation. Using the same virtual scene, the 3D ring model is overlaid such that the commissural points of ring and annulus coincide, following the recommendations from Carpentier (see section 1.2). Different ring models from the set of 14 digitized annuloplasty rings can be selected and adjusted in commercially available sizes. Additional quantitative information about the ring or annulus model can be rendered into the scene such as the transverse or septolateral diameter, circumference or area of the annulus, aiding in the ring selection procedure. A color transfer function can be applied to the surface of the ring to indicate regions of larger displacement between ring and annulus (green: low displacement, red: high displacement) [4]. Arrows can be displayed to reveal the relation between the relative positions of ring and anatomical structure.

2.4 Evaluation

The evaluation has been divided into two parts: (1) the evaluation of the reliability of suture detection and (2) the accuracy of pose estimation. For the first task, we manually marked the entry points of the green sutures into the tissue on 12 randomly selected endoscopic frames from the scene, which forms our ground truth. Since the entry point is not really a single point, but a larger

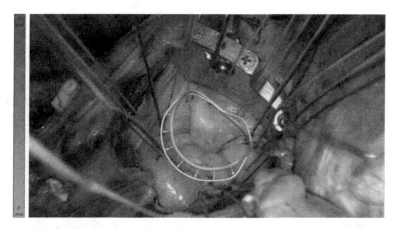

Fig. 4. Augmented reality-enhanced endoscopic image for annuloplasty ring selection. The white curve depicts the patient-specific annulus segmented from TEE images. The color-coded curve represents the virtual ring implant.

region of several pixels, a suture detection was considered successful, if the tip of the suture was detected within a maximum distance of 10 pixels from the ground truth. Every matching candidate is considered as true positive (TP), and every candidate that does not match a ground truth region is called a false positive (FP). If a ground truth region is not matched by any detected suture point, it is called a false negative (FN). The detection performance is described by the true-positive rate (TPR) and the false-positive rate (FPR) defined as $TPR = |TP|/(|TP| + |FN|)$ and $FPR = |FP|/(|TP| + |FP|)$. Additionally, since we want to detect the circular annulus, we evaluated the mean Euclidean distance and standard deviation of the absolute difference in $r(\phi)$ between a spline through the ground truth points and a spline through the detected points.

For the second task, the determined pose of the 3D model has been reprojected onto the image. In an ideal world (with the heart not deforming interoperatively), the reprojected points should coincide with the 2D suture points. To determine the pose estimation error, we calculate the distance between the reprojected points and the detected 2D suture points, in the following called backprojection error. We also compute the fiducial registration error, which we define as the mean distance between the 3D correspondence sets (ray points and object points) after the final iteration.

3   Results

In total, 139 ground truth suture entry points have been evaluated. The suture detection had a $TPR = 0.583$ and a $FPR = 0.314$ with $TP = 81$, $FP = 37$ and $FN = 58$. The mean Euclidean distance between the reconstructed ground truth spline and the spline connecting the detected end points was 19.4 ± 6.6 pixels. The mean fiducial registration error between the 3D points on the projection rays and the points on the 3D annulus contour was 4.9 ± 1.9 mm after 1000 iterations. The mean backprojection error was 12.1 ± 5.9 pixels.

4   Discussion and Conclusion

The presented work describes an augmented reality application which has the potential to be deployed into clinical routine, since no additional hardware is neccessary. The aim is to aid the surgeon intraoperatively in providing decision support for annuloplasty ring selection during MV reconstruction.

Information about suture placement is probably a valuable information on its own, because it influences the geometry of the valve after repair. We used the suture information for determination of the anatomical position of the annulus in the image frame. In our application, the system already works with a relatively low TPR of the end point detection, because the pose estimation step can handle this lack of information, resulting in a mean 2D reprojection error of 12.1 pixels. We showed that our pipeline is capable of detecting sufficient features to reconstruct the oval arrangement of the sutures without large outliers (mean Euclidean distance of spline to ground truth spline is 19.4 pixels).

We expected to observe a certain error in the reprojection of the 3D annulus model, since the intraoperative anatomy of the cardioplegic heart generally differs from the anatomy captured in the functional TEE ultrasound image. This implies that the 2D suture points in the endoscopic image do not exactly depict the 3D annulus object points as determined in the ultrasound image. However, the error is small and we do not see a huge drawback for this augmented reality application. We selected a systolic time step from the cardiac cycle, because this state is assumed to be the most similar to the intraoperative state of the annulus.

The intermediate step of visually assessing the valve using traditional sizer instruments could be overcome by this computer-assisted method. The sizing itself and especially switching between several sizer instruments is time consuming. Therefore, we can envisage an acceleration of the procedure. Moreover, instrument sterilisation becomes superfluous. Another drawback of the traditional sizing method is that the relation between ring and patient-specific annulus becomes only obvious after implantation. Our computer-based system provides a preview of the prosthesis in its later environment. The surgeon gets a direct visual impression about the resulting orifice of the MV which would result from implantation of the selected ring. Likewise, more elaborate quantifications on the patient-specific annulus and the ring prosthesis can be obtained in comparison to the traditional planar sizing instrument.

The red color-coding on the ring indicates regions of high distances between the selected prosthesis and annulus, as shown in figure 4. This information might help in repairing asymmetric dilated annuli, where the ends of the sutures should be placed in closer proximity on the ring. Thus, our proposed system is capable of assisting in the next surgical steps of ring selection and, additionally, in suture placement on the ring after suture placement on the annulus.

An evaluation of the proposed pipeline on a large collection of endoscopic and ultrasound data has still to be performed. Furthermore, continuity information about the movement of the sutures will be integrated into the algorithm to make it more robust against outliers. Tracking the suture points over time after their initial detection with the proposed pipeline might be a viable solution to allow real time processing.

Acknowledgements. This research was carried out with the support of the German Research Foundation (DFG) within project B01, *SFB/TRR 125 Cognition-Guided Surgery.*

References

1. Bothe, W., Miller, D.C., Doenst, T.: Sizing for mitral annuloplasty: Where does science stop and voodoo begin? Ann. Thorac. Surg. 95(4), 1475–1483 (2013)
2. Carpentier, A.: Cardiac valve surgery–the "French correction". J. Thorac. Cardiovasc. Surg. 86(3), 323–337 (1983)
3. Carpentier, A., Adams, D.H., Filsoufi, F.: Carpentier's Reconstructive Valve Surgery. Elsevier Health Sciences (2010)
4. Graser, B., Seitel, M., Al-Maisary, S., Grossgasteiger, M., et al.: Computer-assisted analysis of annuloplasty rings. In: Bildverarbeitung für die Medizin 2013, pp. 75–80. Springer (2013)
5. Graser, B., Wald, D., Al-Maisary, S., Grossgasteiger, M., et al.: Using a shape prior for robust modeling of the mitral annulus on 4D ultrasound data. Int. J. Comput. Assist. Radiol. Surg., 1–10 (2013)
6. Horn, B.: Closed-form solution of absolute orientation using unit quaternions. Journal of the Optical Society of America A 4(4), 629–642 (1987)
7. Maisano, F., Skantharaja, R., Denti, P., et al.: Mitral annuloplasty. Multimedia Manual of Cardio-Thoracic Surgery, 2009(0918):mmcts.2008.003640 (2009)
8. Maurer, C., Qi, R., Raghavan, V.: A Linear Time Algorithm for Computing Exact Euclidean Distance Transforms of Binary Images in Arbitrary Dimensions. IEEE Trans. Pattern Anal. Mach. Intell. 25(2), 265–270 (2003)
9. Nolden, M., Zelzer, S., Seitel, A., Wald, D., et al.: The Medical Imaging Interaction Toolkit: challenges and advances: 10 years of open-source development. Int. J. Comput. Assist. Radiol. Surg. 8(4), 607–620 (2013)
10. Rosenhahn, B., Krüger, N., Rabsch, T., Sommer, G.: Tracking with a novel pose estimation algorithm. In: Klette, R., Peleg, S., Sommer, G. (eds.) RobVis 2001. LNCS, vol. 1998, pp. 9–18. Springer, Heidelberg (2001)
11. Sato, Y., Nakajima, S., Atsumi, H., Koller, T., et al.: 3D multi-scale line filter for segmentation and visualization of curvilinear structures in medical images. In: Troccaz, J., Mösges, R., Grimson, W.E.L. (eds.) CVRMed-MRCAS 1997. LNCS, vol. 1205, pp. 213–222. Springer, Heidelberg (1997)
12. Shi, J., Tomasi, C.: Good features to track. In: Proceedings of the IEEE Conference on Computer Vision and Pattern Recognition, pp. 593–600 (1994)
13. Sommer, C., Straehle, C., Kothe, U., Hamprecht, F.A.: Ilastik: Interactive learning and segmentation toolkit. In: IEEE International Symposium on Biomedical Imaging (ISBI), pp. 230–233 (2011)
14. Zhang, Z.: A flexible new technique for camera calibration. IEEE Trans. Pattern Anal. Mach. Intell. 22(11), 1330–1334 (2000)

A Framework for Semi-automatic Fiducial Localization in Volumetric Images

Dénes Ákos Nagy[1], Tamás Haidegger[2], and Ziv Yaniv[1]

[1] The Sheikh Zayed Institute for Pediatric Surgical Innovation, Children's National Health System, Washington, DC 20010, USA
[2] Antal Bejczy Center for Intelligent Robotics, Obuda University, Hungary
ZYaniv@childrensnational.org

Abstract. Fiducial localization in volumetric images is a common task performed by image-guided navigation and augmented reality systems. These systems often rely on fiducials for image-space to physical-space registration, or as easily identifiable structures for registration validation purposes. Automated methods for fiducial localization in volumetric images are available. Unfortunately, these methods are not generalizable as they explicitly utilize strong a priori knowledge, such as fiducial intensity values in CT, or known spatial configurations as part of the algorithm. Thus, manual localization has remained the most general approach, readily applicable across fiducial types and imaging modalities. The main drawbacks of manual localization are the variability and accuracy errors associated with visual localization. We describe a semi-automatic fiducial localization approach that combines the strengths of the human operator and an underlying computational system. The operator identifies the rough location of the fiducial, and the computational system accurately localizes it via intensity based registration, using the mutual information similarity measure. This approach is generic, implicitly accommodating for all fiducial types and imaging modalities. The framework was evaluated using five fiducial types and three imaging modalities. We obtained a maximal localization accuracy error of 0.35 mm, with a maximal precision variability of 0.5 mm.

1 Introduction

Surgical augmented reality and image-guided navigation systems aim to enhance the clinician's ability to interpret the underlying surgical scene observed via intra-operative imaging. This is most often achieved by registering high quality pre-operative images to the intra-operative physical setting [2,20]. Registration is typically performed using a rigid paired-point approach as it has an analytic solution [7]. Fiducials are localized in the pre-operative image and intra-operatively localized using a tracked calibrated pointer.

Performing paired point, rigid or non-rigid, registration in a robust, accurate, and precise manner is a key task in navigation and guidance systems, aligning image-space and physical-space. It is also in wide spread use in research laboratories where it serves as a means for estimating a ground truth transformation

C.A. Linte et al. (Eds.): AE-CAI 2014, LNCS 8678, pp. 138–148, 2014.

for evaluating results obtained with novel image-to-image or image-to-physical registration methods [4,3,8].

The nomenclature describing the various errors in paired point registration was introduced in [11], defining the three relevant quantities: Fiducial Localization Error (FLE), Fiducial Registration Error (FRE), and Target Registration Error (TRE). Thus, to minimize the TRE we need to reduce FLE. In other words, we want to precisely and accurately localize the fiducials in image-space.

We next present, in chronological order, existing approaches to fiducial localization described in the literature.

The simplest form of localization is for a human operator to visually localize the fiducials in the volumetric image. This approach is common due to its simplicity and the robustness of the human operator to variations in imaging modalities and fiducial geometries and appearances. Studies that report the values of image-space FLE that can be expected in the clinical setting using skin adhesive fiducials were described in [18,13]. According to these reports, typical values for FLE in the image domain are in the range of 0.82.3 mm. These depend upon the imaging modality, MR or CT, associated spatial resolution, and the fiducial type in use. A study designed to evaluate FLE using a custom phantom with divot fiducials and manual localization in CT reported FLE values in the range of 0.4-0.8 mm [9]. Most likely these lower values are associated with the use of CT and the specific fiducial choice.

Possibly the first automated method was presented in [17]. Cylindrical markers with known dimension are automatically localized in CT and MR. The algorithm is comprised of two parts identification of potential fiducial locations and fiducial localization. The first part identifies potential fiducial locations using thresholding and morphological operations. The second part determines if a candidate is indeed a fiducial by comparing the size and shape of the connected component and the known fiducial size and radius. The fiducial is localized using the intensity weighted centroid of the connected component. It should be noted that in practice MR and CT are treated differently, with modality specific steps described as part of the algorithm. The method was shown to have a 1.4% false positive identification error rate localizing 168 fiducials.

In [6] an automated algorithm for localizing fiducials in CT and MR is presented. The method first identifies potential fiducial locations using the mathematical morphology top-hat operator; then, assuming no false negatives, it removes candidates that are too close to each other based on the intensity values in the candidate regions. Finally, localization is performed using the intensity weighted centroid of the region. The method was only evaluated on a single CT scan of a phantom with eight cylindrical fiducials. All fiducials were localized, but given the sample size it is unclear if this method can indeed deal with various fiducial types and modalities.

In [12] donut shaped fiducials are automatically localized in CT. A fixed intensity threshold is used to identify the patient and fiducials, this is followed by morphological operations that result in identification of connected components that are deemed to be fiducial locations. Each fiducial is localized using the intensity weighted centroid of the connected component. The method was shown to have less than 5% false negative and 2.3% false positive identification error rate localizing 25 fiducials.

In [14] a method based on template matching on the edge detection results of CT or MR is presented. The method is customized for donut fiducials that are commonly used by clinical systems. The method successfully identified fiducials in two CT and five MR data sets. Evaluation of the localization accuracy is not provided.

A method designed for automatic donut fiducial detection on cranial images is described [1]. The method is based on identification of fiducial corner points in the 2D edge detected result obtained from CT or MR. The corners are clustered via K-means and a polynomial curve is fit to the corner points. The center point of the curves is defined as the fiducial location. The method successfully localized fiducials in 56 CTs with a difference of 0.5 mm or less from a manually defined ground truth. On 66 MR images the method only failed twice.

Another method designed for automatic donut fiducial detection in cranial images is described in [16]. This method takes the 3D nature of the data into account and uses a local 2D height map based template matching approach to identify fiducial locations. First, the head surface is segmented from the CT or MR volume using a threshold. Then at each surface voxel location the distance between the surface and the plane defined by the voxel and the vector connecting it to the center of the volume/head is estimated. This local height map is then compared to the fiducial's height map. If the difference between the two height maps is less than a threshold this is a potential fiducial. All potential fiducial locations are clustered using a nearest neighbor approach. The marker is then localized by taking the candidate location whose height map is most similar to the fiducial's height map. The method was evaluated using 15 CT, and 10 MRI data sets. In CT(MR) 69/75(47/52) fiducials were accurately localized.

A more recent method for automatic spherical fiducial localization in cranial CT images is described in [5]. The method is specific to CT as the intensity value of the fiducials is used as part of the localization approach. A set of surfaces is obtained from the CT using the marching cubes algorithm. The surface that corresponds to the head is removed and the remaining surfaces are categorized as fiducial or not based on the known fiducial geometry by comparing the surface's bounding box size to the expected size and the Hausdorff distance between the surface and a sphere positioned at the center of the bounding box. Once a surface is classified as a fiducial its location is estimated as the centroid of the surface vertices. The method was evaluated on clinical data with 211/233 fiducials accurately localized.

It should be noted that each of these localization methods was evaluated using a single fiducial type, with some of the algorithms customized to the specific fiducial geometry or the anatomical structure on which they are attached, such as the head. In all of these algorithms the fiducial configuration is arbitrary. This necessitates visual confirmation as none of these algorithms can guarantee success, all fiducials correctly localized without any false positives. A strong constraint, that allows one to dispense with visual confirmation, is the use of a known fiducial configuration.

We propose to use a common framework for semi-automatic fiducial localization that is not tailored to a specific fiducial. The approach combines the strengths of a human operator and an underlying computational system. The operator performs a recognition task, identifying the presence of a fiducial in a rough location, and the computational system accurately localizes it. We next describe our approach in detail.

2   Materials and Methods

Our framework for fiducial localization in volumetric images is a natural extension of manual localization and thus fits within the existing clinical practice. We formulate fiducial localization as a multi-modality intensity based rigid registration task. Fiducials are modeled as volumetric images. In our case we use binary volumes, although other intensity models are readily accommodated by our framework. A straightforward method for creating additional fiducial models is to acquire a high quality volumetric scan of the new fiducial and accurately localize it in that image.

To localize a fiducial in an image the operator identifies the rough fiducial location in the image by clicking anywhere inside it, we then register the fiducial model to the image with the indicated location serving as the initial translational part of a rigid transformation. As most often fiducials represent a single point, we require that the origin of the model fiducial image be located at this point. Thus, the translational part of the transformation obtained by intensity based registration becomes the point we seek.

The fiducial model is registered locally, with the region of interest defined to be twice the size of the fiducial model image diameter. This ensures that even if the operator identified the fiducial's edge the whole fiducial is contained in our region of interest. The rigid transformation is parameterized using three translation components, with rotation represented by the three Euler angles. We use the Nelder-Mead downhill simplex as our optimizer, as it does not require the computation of derivatives. Given that our goal is to localize the fiducials in all modalities using the same framework, we use mutual information as our similarity measure [15,10].

As is well known, the success of iterative registration algorithms is highly dependent on initialization. In our case initialization only provides a constraint on the location of the fiducial and not its orientation. This is a critical issue, as registration will most likely fail if a correct registration means that the fiducial model image should be rotated by 180° around one of its axes, which is not uncommon. We therefor associate a set of rotations with each fiducial model. Together with the location these define a set of initializations used to localize the fiducial. It should be noted that this set of orientations is dependent on the fiducial geometry. In case of a spherical fiducial there is only one rotation, the identity. Other commonly used fiducials such as the Beekly PinPoint (Beekley

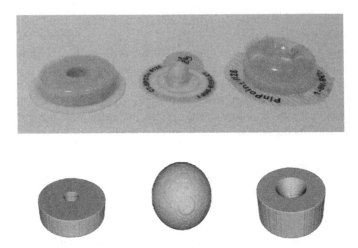

Fig. 1. Fiducial types used for framework evaluation: (top) physical fiducials (bottom) surface representation of the binary fiducial models

Corp.,CT, USA) or the IZI multi modality markers (IZI Medical Products, MD, USA), shown in Figure 1, do require multiple orientations. As these two fiducial types are symmetric around one axis, they each have six orientations associated with them. We thus perform multiple registrations starting from the set of initializations defined by the fiducial geometry. The transformation obtained by the registration with the optimal similarity measure value is taken as the correct one.

An interesting issue with the IZI multi-modality markers is that they have two sets of symmetry planes. The more problematic one is due to the fact that the part that is adhered to the patient is symmetric to the top of this cylindrical fiducial. If we only modeled the fiducial this symmetry cannot be resolved. We therefor break the symmetry by slightly enlarging the image model so that it incorporates the fiducial, and above the fiducial an empty region. This matches the physical setup where the region above the fiducial contains air.

Our framework uses the following parameter values. For Mutual Information estimation we use 24 histogram bins and 0.4 of the pixels of the fiducial image. We set the function convergence tolerance to 0.001, the parameters convergence tolerance to 0.25 and the maximum number of iterations to 200.

3   Experimental Evaluation

To evaluate our fiducial localization framework we used the following set of fiducials: (1) 4 mm diameter sphere; (2) 6 mm diameter sphere; (3) multi modality markers from IZI, referred to as donut fiducials; (4) the PinPoint multi modality markers from Beekly, referred to as cone fiducials; and (5) conical divot markers. Figure 1 shows a subset of these and corresponding surface models. The fiducials

Table 1. Number of localized fiducials per modality, number of scans in parenthesis. Top part of the table are phantom data sets, bottom part are clinical data sets. Five different forms of fiducials were localized, for a total of 95 unique localizations.

modality	sphere 4 mm	sphere 6 mm	donut	cone	divot
CT	5(1)	-	5 (1)	5(1)	12 (1)
CBCT	13(3)	20(4)	-	-	-
MR	-	-	-	5(1)	-
CT	-	-	9(1)	-	-
MR	-	-	15(2)	9(1)	-

were imaged using three modalities: CT, MR and Cone-Beam CT (CBCT). In some cases the images are of phantoms and in others clinical images. The data used in this evaluation study is described in Table 1.

The framework's precision was evaluated exhaustively. All of the fiducials are roughly localized in all data sets. We then perform an initial localization using the operator provided location as described above. The output of this localization serves as the input for our precision evaluation. We construct a set of concentric spheres centered on this point with each sphere having a radius 0.5 mm larger than the previous one. We randomly selected points on each of the spheres serving as user input for our framework. We quantify precision as the distance between the initial point used to construct the set of spheres and the result of each of the registrations.

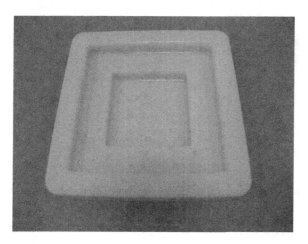

Fig. 2. Plastic phantom with divots whose location is known with high accuracy

Evaluating accuracy is a non-trivial task, as the true fiducial location is never known. Instead we use common surrogates. In our case, we localized all spherical fiducials using the weighted intensity centroid (implementation found online, ground truth for fiducial localization in CBCT [19]). We take the result of this approach as the reference fiducial location. In addition, we also designed a phantom with a dozen divot holes at known locations and used a highly accurate 3D printer, Objet500 Connex from Stratasys, to print it. Figure 2 shows this phantom. Finally, on two clinical data sets we used a common strategy for obtaining a reference localization; we had multiple, in our case five, operators manually localize donut fiducials and used the mean of this localization as the reference fiducial location.

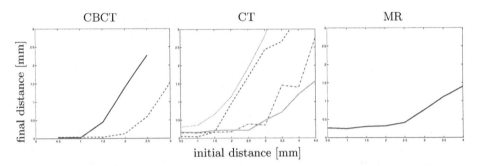

Fig. 3. Precision using phantom data. Each point on the graphs represents the average of 100 initializations. In CBCT we used 4 mm diameter spheres (continuous, blue, line) and 6 mm diameter spheres (dashed, green, line). In CT we used 4 mm spheres (dashed, green, line), cones (continuous, cyan, line), divots (dotted, blue, line) and donuts (dash-dot, red, line). In MR we used cones.

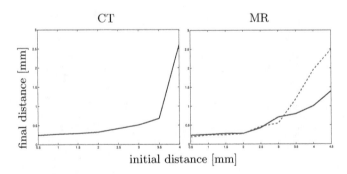

Fig. 4. Precision using clinical data. Each point on the graphs represents the average of 100 initializations. In CT we used donut fiducials. In MR we used cone fiducials (continuous, blue, line) and donut (dashed, green, line).

4   Results

Our evaluation results for precision, both for phantom and clinical data, show a precision of less than 0.5 mm for all fiducial types. The breakdown point in precision occurs once the initialization is far enough from the actual fiducial location so that the whole fiducial is not encompassed by our region of interest. As the region of interest is determined by the fiducial size we observed that the breakdown point for larger fiducials was further away from their actual location, as is expected. Figures 3 and 4 summarize our experiments for phantom and clinical data.

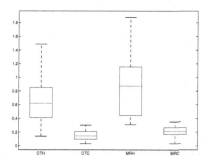

Fig. 5. Precision of fiducial localization in mm. Donut fiducials localized in clinical CT and MR (CTH/MRH-manual, CTC/MRC-semi-automated). The precision of the semi-automated method is clearly better.

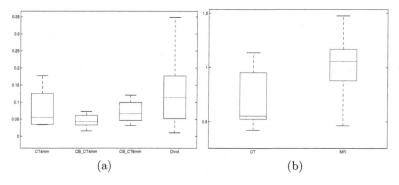

(a)   (b)

Fig. 6. Accuracy evaluation results in mm, (a) using phantom data and (b) using donut fiducials on clinical data

While our results show that the proposed approach is highly precise, it is interesting to compare this approach to the human operator's precision. To compare the two, we took the manual "accurate" localizations used to define a ground truth on the clinical data. This illustrates the inter-observer variability and associated precision. We compare this to the variability associated with the proposed approach when the input is a rough localization. Figure 5 illustrates the higher precision of our method.

Having established that our framework is precise, we now look at its accuracy. Our framework obtained results with a maximal error of 0.35 mm on phantom data. This is in comparison to the ground truth obtained by using another semi-automated localization approach, intensity weighted centroid, and to a ground truth known from phantom construction. On clinical data our framework obtained results with a maximal error of 1.5 mm. Figure 6 summarizes our accuracy evaluation. The accuracy results on the clinical data are significantly lower. Most likely this is due to the quality of our reference gold standard, averaging of multiple manual localizations. This observation is supported by the low precision exhibited by manual localization as seen in Figure 5.

5   Discussion and Conclusions

We have presented a semi-automated framework for fiducial localization. The framework was evaluated for precision and accuracy using three fiducial geometries, sphere, cone, and donut. In all data sets all of the fiducials were accurately localized. Our approach is based on the robustness provided by the human operator, readily identifying the presence and rough location of fiducials. Once a fiducial is identified the registration based approach accurately and precisely localizes it.

While our approach is only semi-automatic, it is clinically acceptable as it is a slight modification of the existing workflow, and places less requirements on the operator. That is, instead of accurate localization the operator need only identify the rough location of the fiducial. In addition, by taking advantage of the robustness of the operator's visual system complex settings are readily accommodated for in an implicit manner, something that is not trivial when proposing fully automated localization schemes. Point in case, we used a clinical CT for evaluation in which the patient's head was in a head rest (Figure 7). None of the human operators was distracted by this, implicitly dealing with

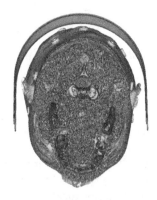

Fig. 7. Volume rendering of cranial CT image used in our evaluation. Note the presence of the head rest.

confounding information which would most likely cause automated methods to fail.

Acknowledgment. We would like to thank Kendall O'Brien for his help with image acquisition, and the following people for their help with the experiments Özgür Güler, Rahul Khare, Reza Monfaredi, Reza Seifabadi, and Emmanuel Wilson.

D. Nagy was supported by a grant from the HungarianAmerican Enterprise Scholarship Fund. T. Haidegger was supported by the Bolyai program of the Hungarian Academy of Sciences.

References

1. Chen, D., Tan, J., Chaudhary, V., Sethi, I.K.: Automatic fiducial localization in brain images. International Journal of Computer Assisted Radiology and Surgery 1(1 suppl.), 45–47 (2006)
2. Cleary, K., Peters, T.M.: Image-guided interventions: technology review and clinical applications. Annu. Rev. Biomed. Eng. 12, 119–142 (2010)
3. Dang, H., Otake, Y., Schafer, S., Stayman, J.W., Kleinszig, G., Siewerdsen, J.H.: Robust methods for automatic image-to-world registration in cone-beam CT interventional guidance. Med. Phys. 39(10), 6484–6498 (2012)
4. Fallavollita, P., Aghaloo, Z.K., Burdette, E.C., Song, D.Y., Abolmaesumi, P., Fichtinger, G.: Registration between ultrasound and fluoroscopy or CT in prostate brachytherapy. Med. Phys. 37(6), 2749–2760 (2010)
5. Fattori, G., Riboldi, M., Desplanques, M., Tagaste, B., Pella, A., Orecchia, R., Baroni, G.: Automated fiducial localization in CT images based on surface processing and geometrical prior knowledge for radiotherapy applications. IEEE Trans. Biomed. Eng. 59(8), 2191–2199 (2012)
6. Gu, L., Peters, T.: 3D automatic fiducial marker localization approach for frameless stereotactic neuro-surgery navigation. In: Yang, G.Z., Jiang, T.-Z. (eds.) MIAR 2004. LNCS, vol. 3150, pp. 329–336. Springer, Heidelberg (2004)
7. Horn, B.K.P.: Closed-form solution of absolute orientation using unit quaternions. Journal of the Optical Society of America A 4(4), 629–642 (1987)
8. Ji, S., Roberts, D.W., Hartov, A., Paulsen, K.D.: Intraoperative patient registration using volumetric true 3D ultrasound without fiducials. Med. Phys. 39(12), 7540–7552 (2012)
9. Liu, W., Ding, H., Han, H., Xue, Q., Sun, Z., Wang, G.: The study of fiducial localization error of image in point-based registration. In: International Conference of the IEEE Engineering in Medicine and Biology Society (EMBC), pp. 5088–5091 (2009)
10. Mattes, D., Haynor, D.R., Vesselle, H., Lewellen, T.K., Eubank, W.: PET-CT image registration in the chest using free-form deformations. IEEE Trans. Med. Imag. 22(1), 120–128 (2003)
11. Maurer, J. C.R., Fitzpatrick, J.M., Wang, M.Y., Galloway Jr., R.L., Maciunas, R.J., Allen, G.S.: Registration of head volume images using implantable fiducial markers. IEEE Trans. Med. Imag. 16(4), 447–462 (1997)
12. Nicolau, S., Garcia, A., Pennec, X., Soler, L., Ayache, N.: An augmented reality system to guide radio-frequency tumour ablation. Comput. Anim. Virtual Worlds 16(1), 1–10 (2005)

13. Shamir, R.R., Joskowicz, L., Spektor, S., Shoshan, Y.: Localization and registration accuracy in image guided neurosurgery: a clinical study. International Journal of Computer Assisted Radiology and Surgery 4(1), 45–52 (2009)
14. Tan, J., Chen, D., Chaudhary, V., Sethi, I.: A template based technique for automatic detection of fiducial markers in 3D brain images. International Journal of Computer Assisted Radiology and Surgery 1, 47–49 (2006)
15. Viola, P., Wells III, W.M.: Alignment by maximization of mutual information. International Journal of Computer Vision 24(2), 137–154 (1997)
16. Wang, M., Song, Z.: Automatic localization of the center of fiducial markers in 3D CT/MRI images for image-guided neurosurgery. Pattern Recognition Letters 30(4), 414–420 (2009)
17. Wang, M.Y., Maurer, J.C.R., Fitzpatrick, J.M., Maciunas, R.J.: An automatic technique for finding and localizing externally attached markers in CT and MR volume images of the head. IEEE Trans. Biomed. Eng. 43(6), 627–637 (1996)
18. Woerdeman, P.A., Willems, P.W., Noordmans, H.J., van der Sprenke, J.W.B.: The effect of repetitive manual fiducial localization on target localization in image space. Neurosurgery 60(2 suppl. 1), ONS-100–ONS-103 (2007)
19. Yaniv, Z.: Localizing spherical fiducials in c-arm based cone-beam CT. Med. Phys. 36(11), 4957–4966 (2009)
20. Yaniv, Z., Cleary, K.: Image-guided procedures: A review. Tech. Rep. CAIMR TR-2006-3, Image Science and Information Systems Center, Georgetown University (April 2006)

Author Index